Socialising the Biomedical Turn in HIV Prevention

Key Issues in Modern Sociology

This series publishes scholarly texts by leading social theorists that give an accessible exposition of the major structural changes in modern societies. The volumes in the series address an academic audience through their relevance and scholarly quality, and connect sociological thought to public issues. The series covers both substantive and theoretical topics, as well as addresses the works of major modern sociologists. The series emphasis is on modern developments in sociology with relevance to contemporary issues such as globalization, warfare, citizenship, human rights, environmental crises, demographic change, religion, postsecularism and civil conflict.

Series Editor

Simon Susen – City University London, UK

Editorial Board

Thomas Cushman – Wellesley College, USA
Peter Kivisto – Augustana College, USA
Rob Stones – University of Western Sydney, Australia
Richard Swedberg – Cornell University, USA
Stephen Turner – University of South Florida, USA
Darin Weinberg – University of Cambridge, UK

Socialising the Biomedical Turn in HIV Prevention

Susan Kippax
and
Niamh Stephenson

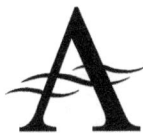

ANTHEM PRESS

Anthem Press
An imprint of Wimbledon Publishing Company
www.anthempress.com

This edition first published in UK and USA 2019
by ANTHEM PRESS
75–76 Blackfriars Road, London SE1 8HA, UK
or PO Box 9779, London SW19 7ZG, UK
and
244 Madison Ave #116, New York, NY 10016, USA

First published in the UK and USA by Anthem Press 2016

British Library Cataloguing-in-Publication Data
A catalogue record for this book is available from the British Library.

ISBN-13: 978-1-78527-125-0 (Pbk)
ISBN-10: 1-78527-125-3 (Pbk)

This title is also available as an e-book.

This book is dedicated to
Robert Ariss, Tim Carrigan and Brett Tindall – three gay men
whose lives and work informed this research,
and who died of AIDS

CONTENTS

FIGURES

TABLES

ACKNOWLEDGEMENTS

The thinking in this book arises from years of collective discussion, debate and research. Many researchers and colleagues working on various aspects of HIV have fuelled our thinking through their encouragement, uptake and reworking of ideas presented here. For this ongoing discussion and provocation we are deeply grateful to Barry Adam, Peter Aggleton, Judith Auerbach, Michael Bartos, Don Baxter, Steve Bell, Alan Brotherton, Liviana Calzavara, Raewyn Connell, June Crawford, Mary Crewe, Ross Duffin, Gary Dowsett, Jeanne Ellard, Sam Friedman, Martin Holt, Paul Kinder, Brent Mackie, Limin Mao, Ann McDonald, Peter McDonald, Ted Myers, Christy Newman, Kane Race, Patrick Rawstorne, Edward Reis, Robert Reynolds, Juliet Richters, Celia Roberts, Marsha Rosengarten, Gary Smith, Paul Van de Ven, Cathy Waldby, Alex Wodak, Heather Worth and Iryna Zablotska. We are also thankful to two readers whose comments have helped to sharpen our argument. And we thank Bryan Turner for encouraging us to write the book.

We are very glad to have had the opportunity to work over elements of this book with students of the Masters in Public Health in the School of Public Health and Community Medicine at the University of New South Wales: their thinking about our approach has helped its development; in particular, thanks to Rosemary Amalo, Hayden Jose, Yves-Laurent Jackson, Evelyn Kwagala and Josephine Okwera Akullu.

The ideas in this book were further developed and challenged by discussions with colleagues whose research involves theorising social relations: Lone Bertelsen, Jayne Bye, Mark Davis, Ros Diprose, Rebecca Edwards, Elisabetta Magnani, Catherine Mills, Anna Munster, Andrew Murphie, Brett Neilson, Dimitris Papadopoulos, Ernst Schraube, Sheila Shaver and kylie valentine.

Also the institutional backing of the University of New South Wales and the collegial support of our colleagues in the Social Policy Research Centre in the Faculty of Arts and Social Sciences and the School of Public Health and Community Medicine in the Faculty of Medicine has been vital in helping us bring this book to publication, as has the ongoing support of Brian Stone and Tej Sood of Anthem Press. We are immensely thankful to Brooke Thompson whose sense of social connectedness gave rise to the cover.

And, finally, a special thanks to Michael Edwards who, in many different ways, supported our work over many, many months with good humour and patience.

Susan Kippax and Niamh Stephenson
December 2015

INTRODUCTION

This book concerns HIV prevention. In it we argue that until the world focuses its attention on the social issues 'both carried and revealed by AIDS' (Fassin, 2007), it is unlikely that HIV transmission will be eradicated or even significantly reduced. The continuing and growing biomedicalisation of HIV prevention, which began in earnest in 1996–1997 after the development of successful HIV treatment and continues with the increasing push to use HIV treatments as prevention, runs the risk of undermining what has been – at least in many countries – a successful prevention response.

Our argument is that at least until such time as biomedicine develops an effective prophylactic vaccine and a cure for the human immunodeficiency virus (HIV), the world must rely on the everyday responses of people and communities to combat HIV. The world must rely on communities and the practices forged by these communities that reduce the risk of HIV transmission (primarily safe sexual and safe drug injection practices); on people's willingness to be identified as infected with HIV (HIV testing practices); and, for people living with HIV, on people's commitment to keep AIDS at bay (HIV treatment practices).

Combating HIV also relies on governments to ensure access to HIV-prevention tools, including condoms and sterile needles and syringes, as well as to biomedical prevention technologies, including those derived from successful antiretroviral treatment (ART) – pre-exposure prophylaxis (PrEP), microbicides and post-exposure prophylaxis (PEP) and male circumcision. It relies on governments to develop robust health infrastructures to support and enable regular HIV testing and to provide access to treatments for those living with HIV. It relies on governments to adopt pragmatic policies that are not deflected by moralistic or conservative ideologies. More broadly, combating HIV depends on civil society resisting HIV stigma and discrimination against those infected and affected by HIV, thereby enabling people and communities to discuss sex and sexuality and drug use in ways that promote safe sexual and drug injection practices.

We take issue with a number of widely held biomedical understandings and positions that are affecting, we believe adversely, an effective HIV-prevention response. Although we touch on a number of such issues in the book, the most central are as follows: First, until there is an efficacious prophylactic vaccine, the search for a magic bullet is misplaced. No one mode of prevention will necessarily be generalisable from one country to another or unchanging from one time to another. What works in Uganda may not work in Australia, and what worked in 2010 may not work in 2020: the responses of peoples and communities to HIV are contingent. Second, somewhat relatedly, effective HIV-prevention interventions do not simply *cause* a reduction in HIV incidence. Rather, effective HIV-prevention programmes reinforce, or produce, responses in people such that safer practices, those that reduce HIV-transmission, become normative. To date, it is in this way that HIV incidence has been reduced. The emergence and sustaining of these 'HIV-reduction responses' depend on a number of factors other than the biological: economic, political, social and psychological.

Third, prevention and treatment are very different from each other – at least until biomedicine produces an effective cure for HIV. The conflation of prevention and treatment, or the insistence that prevention and treatment are on some sort of linear continuum is misleading. While it makes sense to combine drugs to treat HIV, it rarely makes sense to combine prevention modes. Few prevention modes are complementary and, indeed, adopting one form of prevention typically rules out another: for example, people who are HIV-negative are highly unlikely to use condoms and to take prophylactic drugs in order to reduce their risk of HIV infection.

Fourth, although biomedicine may demonstrate that a particular prevention technology is efficacious – that is, it reduces HIV transmission under ideal conditions in individuals – this does not mean that it will be effective, that is, will reduce HIV incidence in populations over time. While it is up to biomedicine to produce efficacious prevention technologies, it is up to social scientists to guide the uptake and use of these efficacious technologies in the real world and to ensure that they are effective and, on the basis of their research, inform prevention and policy responses. It is not the case that an efficacious prevention method will work simply because public health officials or clinicians tell people to embrace them.

An effective response to HIV demands social change and transformation, and social change is complex, emergent, context-dependent and likely to take some time. Our focus is on people understood as 'social beings' (Harré, 1979), on their social relations and practices, and on the ways in which such practices both reproduce and occasionally transform society. We discuss the social and cultural factors that have produced effective HIV prevention and the biomedical understandings and accompanying rhetoric that, we believe, have undermined them. Social and cultural factors are not 'barriers' (a term often used in biomedicine) to effective prevention; rather, they are what need to be engaged with and embraced for prevention to work and be sustained.

Part I of the book, Effective HIV Prevention, examines some of the myriad HIV epidemics affecting various parts of the world, and – through the analysis of two case studies – interrogates what we know about HIV prevention that works. In Chapter 1 we present a summary of the current picture of HIV and its global spread, and the changes in HIV incidence over time. We focus on a small number of countries, in particular, those with different HIV transmission risks and rates, and raise a number of questions with regard to these differences – questions the remainder of the book addresses. What factors have led to the global decline in HIV incidence? What accounts for the differences between countries and regions in the patterning of HIV epidemics? What has led to the current increases in HIV in many countries? In a few words: What works, and what undermines what works?

In Chapter 2 we detail the HIV prevention responses of Uganda. We argue that by allowing those at risk a public voice and thus enabling people to respond collectively to the threat of HIV, Ugandans – at least initially – responded successfully to HIV. As we document, acknowledging and respecting the cultural and social understandings of peoples and communities allowed a robust HIV-prevention response. Although it is difficult to attribute the reduction in HIV incidence to any one particular prevention response, the picture we paint with respect to Uganda's early success in reducing HIV transmission points to the very important role of collectives and the relations and talk between people: a 'social vaccine'.

The sexual practices of people in Uganda continue to be transformed, as we demonstrate with regard to the recent increases in HIV. The once-effective prevention response has faltered, and we raise a number of questions with reference to these recent increases in HIV transmission. We hypothesise that the move to a moral and increasingly biomedical discourse has played a major role in the recent increases in HIV transmission.

In Chapter 3 we turn to Australia to demonstrate what a successful HIV-prevention response looks like. Australia's early response was in many ways very similar to the Ugandan one, although these two countries are very different and have very different HIV epidemics. What is similar in both countries is the central role of a 'social vaccine' in their initial robust response. This response has weakened, and in Australia at present there is growing concern about increasing HIV incidence.

In Part II, Social Transformation, we examine the disjuncture between hegemonic ways of approaching HIV prevention and what is known about effective prevention. We outline the conceptual tools necessary to understand, support and develop effective prevention – concepts that enable the interrogation of the specific social practices entailed in the differing responses of communities to HIV. We begin in Chapter 4 by turning to the biomedical. We document the way in which the HIV story has been, and continues to be, told with reference to the biomedical. Even though the available evidence demonstrates that the global decline in HIV incidence was a function of changes in the sexual and injecting practices of people rather than the result of biomedical interventions, the story is essentially one of biomedical advances. Prevention is to a large degree missing, unless it is deemed biomedical. Although bodies such as the Global HIV Prevention Working Group have acknowledged the role of communities in HIV-prevention responses, the reports from bodies such as the World Health Organisation (WHO) and, more recently, the Joint United Nations Programme on HIV/AIDS (UNAIDS), privilege the biomedical. Using and extending a UNAIDS timeline, we demonstrate the dominance of biomedicine and its increase over time, especially since 1996 with the development of ART and with the push to biomedical prevention in the form of prophylactic drugs (pre-exposure prophylaxis (PrEP) or microbicides) or as 'treatment as prevention' (TasP), which began in the early 2000s. This biomedical dominance is also evident in the ways in which evidence is understood and its 'quality' assessed. This in turn affects the funding policies of bodies such as the National Institutes of Health (NIH), the Bill & Melinda Gates Foundation (the Gates Foundation) and the Global Fund to Fight AIDS, Tuberculosis and Malaria (the Global Fund), with the bulk of funding going to biomedicine or to prevention interventions that take a biomedical approach.

In Chapter 5 we address some of the concepts used in biomedicine. We explore the concept of 'risk' and the concept of 'vulnerability' with reference to the 'risk' behaviours of individuals and the 'vulnerability' of populations. We address HIV testing, especially in relation to counselling, and their roles in prevention in the clinic, and the way in which the 'rational subject' is positioned as the agent of change. As understood within biomedicine, individuals are rational and act sensibly on the basis of public health information to avoid risk, unless they are unable to do so because they are vulnerable. Prevention is reduced to developing interventions that are deemed effective in convincing people to do 'the right thing' as defined by public health or, for the vulnerable, to developing interventions that reduce their vulnerability – although, understandably, such prevention interventions are not common. While vulnerability introduces the notion of the social, it tends to do so in terms of social structures, which render the individual passive and unable to act.

In Chapter 6 we offer an alternative to the biomedical paradigm and argue that the practices of communities are central, both to the transmission of HIV and to its reduction, if not eradication. In particular, we focus on the concept of 'practice' and the ways in which collectives (networks of connected people) can and do act to transform society. With reference to the examples of Uganda and Australia (Chapters 2 and 3) we argue that we need a social narrative to replace, or at the very least complement, the biomedical one. A narrative that enables people to act together to protect themselves and others.

In Chapter 7, through the lens of 'treatment as prevention' (TasP), we conclude by arguing that what has gone awry is biomedicine's takeover of prevention. We make some suggestions as to how HIV prevention might be put back on track by engaging with communities and focusing on the social relationships between people and their social practices. HIV prevention involves the practices that produce, reproduce and transform the social worlds in which people live. Practice is central to our devising – as community members and scientists – effective HIV-prevention responses: responses that differ from region to region, from community to community, from social context to context, and change over time. Efforts to prevent HIV are essentially efforts to change society. While acknowledging that biomedical and social scientists work within different paradigms, we need to understand each other's points of view and work together.

Part I

EFFECTIVE HIV PREVENTION

Chapter 1

MAPPING A SOCIAL DISEASE

As the Joint United Nations Programme on HIV/AIDS (UNAIDS) annual country reports demonstrate, there is not one HIV epidemic but many (UNAIDS, 2014a, 2104b).[1] There are differences in the patterning of HIV prevalence and HIV incidence, in HIV-transmission routes and also in terms of HIV-prevention responses and treatment uptake, all of which vary from country to country and from region to region. There is no singular HIV epidemic: the patterning is local and particular. For example, HIV prevalence ranges from zero in Nauru, a small island in the Pacific that currently has no case of HIV/AIDS, to Swaziland, a country in southern Africa that has one of the world's highest HIV prevalence rates: 31 per cent among adults aged 18–49 years (2014b), a rate that has not changed significantly since 2001 (Whiteside & Strauss, 2014). Because there is not one epidemic, the promise of one 'silver bullet' HIV-prevention strategy is illusory. Rather, we argue here that understanding what kinds of HIV-prevention efforts work, and how they work, demands engaging with the specificities and contingencies of particular epidemics. Understanding and enabling an effective HIV-prevention response demands input from social scientists.

A Brief Review of HIV/AIDS

AIDS was first documented in the United States among gay and other homo-sexually active men in 1981 and, although not identified until later, it was also affecting people in that country who injected drugs. However, it is now clear that long before its identification in the United States – and perhaps as early as the 1920s – AIDS was taking a toll on people in Africa, the majority of whom were heterosexual. Since that time HIV, the human immunodeficiency virus that causes AIDS, has spread from a few widely scattered 'hot spots' to virtually every country in the world. Globally, in 2013 between 32.2 and 37.2 million people were living with HIV, although since 2001 new infections have fallen by 38 per cent (UNAIDS, 2014a).

High prevalence (the proportion of the population living with HIV in a given year) is associated with 'generalised' epidemics, where the major route of transmission is vaginal sexual intercourse in the 'general' (heterosexual) population, while in 'concentrated' epidemics HIV is transmitted primarily through anal intercourse among gay and other homosexually active men, or via injecting practices among people who inject drugs, as well as between sex workers and their clients. Concentrated epidemics, in which HIV is limited in the main to the above sub-populations of people, tend to have lower HIV prevalence rates.

The majority of people living with HIV acquired the disease during their adult years, most as a result of engaging in sexual (primarily vaginal and anal intercourse) and drug injection practices, both profoundly social practices related to intimacy and pleasure. HIV is also transmitted from HIV-infected mothers to their children when giving birth and breastfeeding. It can also be transmitted by the use of contaminated blood or blood products, although most countries have now secured their blood supplies.

The advent of effective treatments in the form of antiretroviral treatments (ART) in 1996 changed the face of the HIV epidemic – in both anticipated and unanticipated ways. ART has meant a huge reduction in AIDS-related deaths among those who have access to these treatments. Although access continues to be a problem in low-income countries, it has increased exponentially in recent years, and in 2013 UNAIDS estimated that around 35 per cent of people living with HIV who were eligible for treatment did not have access to ART (WHO, 2013a). As a result of ART, the number of people dying of AIDS-related causes fell to between 1.4 to 1.7 million in 2013 (UNAIDS, 2014a), down from a peak of between 2.2 to 2.6 million in 2005, which means that globally HIV prevalence has grown and will continue to grow. ART enables the majority of people living with HIV to have reasonably normal lives as long as they continue to adhere to the treatment regimen – and they need to do so for the rest of their lives. There is concern about the long-term impact of treatments and evidence that many stop taking ART. A recent estimate (WHO, 2013a) based on 23 countries found that around 28 per cent of those on ART stop taking their medication after five years, many doing so because they no longer feel ill. Similarly, there are some people, although far fewer, who resist taking up treatment as they do not feel ill. Notwithstanding the challenges of providing access to treatment and of the issues related to uptake and adherence, treatment in the form of ART, although not a cure, has meant that the vast majority of people with HIV live with a manageable chronic disease and no longer face an almost certain early death.

Furthermore, as recently demonstrated by Vernazza et al. (2008) and Cohen et al. (2011), because ART reduces the viral load of those living with HIV, it reduces the risk of HIV transmission to others with whom they have sex or share injection equipment. It therefore has a prevention benefit, and this fact has informed a prevention strategy referred to as 'treatment as prevention' (TasP). HIV incidence (the number of new HIV infections in a population in a given year) has fallen and continues to fall. Worldwide, 2.1 million people became newly infected in 2013, a drop of 38 per cent since 2001, and in the same time period new infections declined among children by 58 per cent as a result of the prevention of mother-to-child transmission programmes (PMTCT) (WHO, 2012, 2014). While some of the decline in HIV incidence may be a function of lowered population viral load and the role of ART in prevention, the decline in HIV incidence began well before the advent of – and widening access to – effective treatment. It is clear that a range of prevention initiatives were and are working – at least in some places and to some degree. With reference to sexual transmission, the use of condoms and reduction in the number of sexual partners have proved successful HIV-prevention strategies, as has the provision of sterile needles and syringes and opioid substitution treatment for those who inject drugs.

Prevention is not simply a biomedical matter and should not be restricted to the clinic. While biomedical prevention strategies such as TasP and male circumcision may reduce the likelihood of HIV transmission, unless we focus attention on the social, as Fassin (2007) has cautioned, we will fail to eradicate HIV. Coates et al. (2008, 676) also note that HIV transmission is a 'social event'. HIV-prevention strategies need to move beyond an attempt to modify the behaviour of individuals who interact with health facilities and are receptive to HIV testing and counselling. Unlike people living with HIV, who are likely to take the advice of public health authorities, those who are uninfected may not be so easily accessed or persuaded. Even if they come forward for frequent HIV testing, they are far less likely than people living with HIV to follow the advice of medical authorities, as we discuss in Chapter 5.

For HIV-prevention strategies, including biomedical strategies, to be effective, they need to acknowledge and engage with the very varied local sexual and drug injection practices of communities and networks of people: community engagement is central to HIV prevention. Effective prevention strategies are rarely generalisable – unlike treatment which, when an efficacious remedy is found and made easily available, almost all individuals benefit from adhering to the treatment regimen.

As we discuss in the remainder of this chapter and in the chapters to follow, countries and regions have different epidemics and have responded in different ways. Certain HIV-prevention strategies are effective for some people and not others, in some places and regions and not others and at some times and not others. HIV is spread by profoundly social practices, and its prevention is aided or thwarted by social practices, which differ from population to population, from region to region and from time period to time period.

Regional Epidemics

Here we indicate some of this variation. Our purpose is not to provide a comprehensive overview of the global epidemics but to indicate some of the known differences and the often very particular HIV epidemics that those involved in prevention across the globe are continually challenged to address.

Sub-Saharan Africa is most severely affected: 24.7 million people were living with HIV in 2013, with nearly 1 in every 20 adults (4.9 per cent) infected, and accounting for around 70 per cent of the people living with HIV worldwide. Notwithstanding the very high prevalence in this generalised form of the HIV epidemic, new infections declined in sub-Saharan Africa by 33 per cent between 2005 and 2013. Treatment coverage is 37 per cent of all people living with HIV, and since 2009 there has been a 43 per cent decline in new infections among children (UNAIDS, 2014a).

Although the regional prevalence of HIV infection is nearly 25 times higher in sub-Saharan Africa than in Asia, 4.8 million people are living with HIV in Asia and the Pacific, and new infections declined by 6 per cent between 2005 and 2013; however, in Indonesia, new HIV infections have risen by 48 per cent – a cause for concern (UNAIDS, 2014a). In Latin America, where 1.6 million people are living with HIV, there was a small decline of 3 per cent in new infections between 2005 and 2013. In the same period, in the Caribbean, with 250,000 people living with HIV, new infections declined by 40 per cent (2014a). In Asia and the Pacific, Latin America and the Caribbean, HIV transmission occurs among 'key populations': men who have sex with men; people who inject drugs; and sex workers and their clients. Treatment coverage varied across these regions, with 33 per cent coverage in Asia and the Pacific, 43 per cent in Latin America and 42 per cent in the Caribbean (2014a).

Going against the recent trend in most countries of relatively stable HIV or declining incidence rates, HIV incidence rose by 5 per cent between 2005 and 2013 in Eastern Europe and Central Asia, which together had 1.1 million people living with HIV. And in the Middle East and North Africa, with 230,000 people living with HIV, incidence rose 7 per cent in this time frame (2014a). Treatment coverage is comparatively low: 21 per cent in Eastern Europe and Central Asia and 11 per cent in the Middle East and North Africa.

With reference to Western and Central Europe and North America, with a combined 2.3 million people living with HIV, although there were dramatic declines in HIV incidence up until about 2000, the HIV epidemic appears to have stabilised in these three areas. Treatment coverage is 51 per cent in these regions. However, there have been small increases in HIV incidence in many gay communities, the major at-risk population, across North America and Europe as well as in Australia and New Zealand.

The differential patterning of HIV infections is a function of many factors, including social, cultural and economic factors that influence the responses of countries to HIV and their ability to provide treatment and also the manner in which they support HIV prevention. Drawing on the UNAIDS Country Progress Reports, augmented where available by other data and reports, we provide some snapshots of several of the different dynamics of HIV epidemics – again, to illustrate the very particular and local nature of the patterning of the HIV epidemics and to raise questions about the nature of effective HIV prevention. We give examples of countries with high HIV prevalence and a more or less stable HIV incidence as well as examples of countries with low HIV prevalence. We also give an example of a country with increasing HIV incidence.

High prevalence countries

The countries with high HIV prevalence rates are, without exception, in southern Africa and, without exception, these counties have generalised epidemics. In some of these high prevalence countries there are also high rates of HIV transmission in particular sub-populations, such as homosexually active men (Baral et al., 2014), but in all of these countries heterosexual transmission is the main route of HIV transmission, and more women than men are infected, especially young women. There are no high-income countries with what is considered to be high HIV prevalence.

We present here the sobering picture of HIV in South Africa and other parts of sub-Saharan Africa. In general, HIV incidence in most countries of sub-Saharan Africa appears to be declining slightly or stable. Data from population-based seroprevalence surveys and sentinel surveillance of pregnant women suggest that the HIV epidemic has reached a plateau in South Africa, with adult HIV prevalence at around 17 per cent. In antenatal care (ANC) clients, HIV prevalence has gradually levelled off at around 30 per cent, after steeply increasing for more than 10 years from 7.6 per cent in 1994 to 29.5 per cent in 2004. In 2010 HIV prevalence was 30.2 per cent among women attending antenatal clinics (see Figure 1.1).

Since the first population-based survey in 2002, national HIV prevalence in the general population has shown an overall downward trend in children (primarily as a result of the scaled-up national PMTCT programme) and a slight upward trend in adults. Among youth aged 15–24 years, HIV prevalence

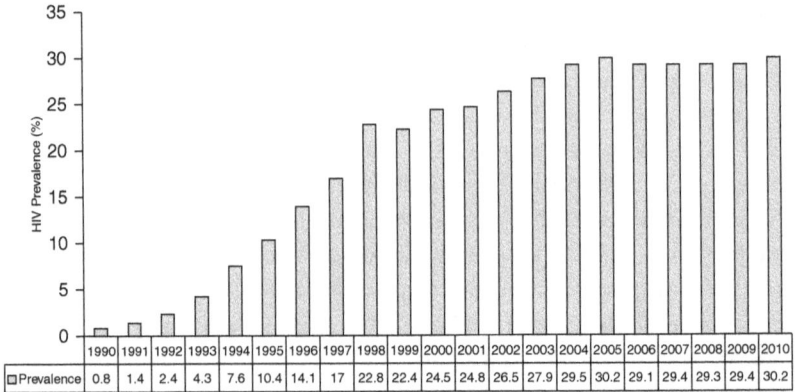

Figure 1.1 HIV prevalence among South African pregnant women aged 15–49 years.
Source: South African Sero-prevalence Survey, 2011, reprinted in South African Country Report to UNAIDS (2012a, 31).

declined from 10.3 per cent in 2005 to 8.7 per cent in 2008 (UNAIDS, 2012a). However, as Leigh et al. (2012) noted, further data are needed to confirm the downward trend, and a recent survey (Shisana et al., 2014) did not show the hoped-for decline among young people.

Part of the reason for these continuing high rates is the decline in condom use over the same periods. In 2012 condom use at last sex decreased to 36.2 per cent, returning to levels similar to those in 2005 of 35.4 per cent, well below the peak of 45.1 per cent in 2008 (Shisana et al., 2014, xxxiv). And although condom use is highest among those aged between 15 and 24 years, these figures are of concern, especially for young women. The HIV incidence rate among female youth aged 15 to 24 years was over four times higher than the incidence rate found in men in this age group (2.5 per cent vs. 0.6 per cent), and young females (15–24) represented nearly a quarter (24.1 per cent) of total new HIV infections. The highest incidence rate in the country in 2012 (4.5 per cent) was among black African women aged 20–34 years (by comparison, adult incidence during the period 2008–2012 was 1.9 per cent). Furthermore, in the context of declining condom use, there has been a slight increase in the proportion of young people reporting 'first sex' before the age of 15 years. There has also been a steady increase over the same time period in the number of respondents who had had more than one partner in the previous 12 months, from 11.5 per cent in 2002 to 18.3 per cent in 2012.

On the basis of their findings – and because of the risk of behavioural disinhibition in the context of the wider availability of ART – Shisana et al. (2014) recommend accelerating social- and behavioural-change communication campaigns. As the authors note in the Executive Summary (2014, xxxix), there was a 'false sense of security observed among some respondents in this survey whereby, based on inaccurate information, some people do not feel that they are at risk of HIV infection'. They also note that the beneficial impact of increased ART coverage on HIV incidence (through viral load reduction in HIV-positive individuals) has been more than offset by the disturbing trends of increased HIV-risk behaviour. They conclude: 'The NSP (National Strategic Plan) for 2012–2016 states as its primary goal a reduction of new infections by at least 50%. In view of our survey findings, this will be extremely difficult to attain given the prevailing transmission dynamics in the country' (2014, xxx).

Botswana, Lesotho, Namibia, Swaziland, Zambia and Zimbabwe also continue to bear the global burden of HIV and AIDS, and all have predominantly heterosexually transmitted epidemics with HIV prevalence over 10 per cent. In two of these countries, Namibia and Zimbabwe, there are signs of a decline in HIV infections (UNAIDS, 2014b) – although in Namibia there are concerns about whether the decline has stalled, and the absence of population-based data means that prevalence can only be estimated through models. There are no indications of declining transmission in Swaziland, Lesotho, Zambia and Botswana (2014b). The 2013 Botswana AIDS Impact Survey (BAIS) (2014b), the fourth of periodic nationally representative behavioural surveys, estimated that 18.5 per cent of the total population was living with HIV, up slightly from 17.6 per cent in 2008. HIV prevalence in the adult population appears to have stabilised at around 24 per cent (Whiteside & Strauss, 2014). With the help of donor funding, Botswana has made significant strides in treating people with HIV. However, it appears that the overwhelming investments in responding to HIV in Botswana have been in the form of treatment provision and, regarding prevention, significant efforts have been made to provide PMTCT, but less has been done to address people's sexual practices. In general, to the extent that the HIV epidemic in these high prevalence countries has stabilised, it has done so at a very high level and appears resistant to the prevention strategies that are currently in play.

Low prevalence countries

Countries with a low HIV prevalence and, up until recently, a reasonably stable HIV incidence include high-income countries with concentrated epidemics that are largely confined to populations of gay and other homosexually active men or, as they are often referred to, men who have sex with men (MSM), and people who inject drugs. Population prevalence in Western Europe in 2011 ranged from 0.02 per cent (in the Czech Republic) to 0.45 per cent (in Portugal). In the same year HIV prevalence was 0.41 per cent in the United States; 0.20 per cent in Canada; 0.15 per cent in the United Kingdom;

0.10 per cent in Australia; 0.06 per cent in New Zealand and 0.01 per cent in Japan (Sullivan et al., 2014). Sullivan et al. (2014) note that in most of these countries, after quite dramatic falls in HIV incidence among MSM up until the early 2000s, incidence increased – the notable exception being Switzerland. It is of concern that almost nowhere in the high-income world is HIV incidence declining among MSM. On the other hand, with the exception of Greece, there appear to have been no increases in HIV incidence among people who inject drugs.

Although it is difficult to give an account of these differences, an examination of trends and responses provide some clues. We take Switzerland as the first example, drawing attention to the early relatively high incidence rate in Switzerland of 42 cases per million inhabitants – the highest HIV incidence in Europe in 1987.[2] The Swiss response to these high figures was swift (Somaini, 2012). Public health experts came together in 1983 with the director of the Federal Office of Public Health (FOPH), the blood supply was secured and the Swiss Cohort Study was established and, together with more recent studies, continues to inform the Swiss strategy by providing invaluable information of the 'state of play' of HIV (Dubois-Arber et al., 1999, 2003). In 1985, the Swiss AIDS Federation was established, comprised of members from the homosexual/gay community, people with haemophilia, people who inject drugs, heterosexuals from high prevalence countries and other affected groups. As the then head of infectious diseases at the FOPH, Somaini, said: 'With this structure, FOPH was much better able to support the many different prevention activities. [...] This was another decision that, almost accidentally, benefited our national response for the long run' (Somaini, 2012, 304). Soon after this partnership was established, all Swiss households were sent a brochure providing information about transmission and how to prevent it, with explicit pictures on how to use a condom. And in 1987 a public campaign, STOP AIDS, was launched to increase public awareness and knowledge about HIV, encourage discussion and promote behavioural changes. Public health initiatives such as the distribution of sterile needles and syringes were also established (Somaini, 306).

This campaign was sustained until replaced by more widely targeted campaigns with the aim of providing everyone living in Switzerland with regular information about HIV/AIDS and ways of protecting against it (UNAIDS, 2014b). Targeted campaigns for MSM, people who inject drugs, heterosexuals from high prevalence countries and other groups at high risk were also undertaken. The FOPH financially supported HIV-prevention activities for MSM and for people who inject drugs and, early in the epidemic, 'Drug Consumption Rooms' and needle and syringe programmes were established in many cantons and cities (Somaini & Grob, 2012). This very public prevention strategy resulted in a decline in HIV incidence, with new infections decreasing because of risk-reduction practices among those groups most at risk. This decline came to an end around the years 2000–2001. In 2002, an incidence increase of 25 per cent was observed. The groups most affected were Swiss MSM and heterosexual persons originating from countries with a high HIV prevalence. Although the total number of new HIV diagnoses remained relatively stable post 2002, the yearly number of positive HIV test results almost doubled among MSM between 2004 and 2008. From 2009, new HIV infections have declined to around 600 per year (down from around 800 per year between 2003 and 2008).

This decline in new HIV infections among MSM in Switzerland, a result of concerted public health campaigns, is a noteworthy exception because in almost all other high-income countries HIV infection rates in this population have increased. In all of them – Denmark, France, Germany, Norway, the Netherlands, Sweden, the United Kingdom, Canada, Australia and New Zealand – the majority of HIV infections occur among MSM, and the general picture in each is similar: declines in HIV infections in MSM occurred between the early 1980s and the end of the 1990s, followed by slight but significant increases that began in the late 1990s and early 2000s.

High-income countries are not the only ones with low HIV prevalence rates. Besides Japan, other countries in East and South East Asia, such as China, Malaysia and Cambodia, also have concentrated epidemics with relatively low HIV prevalence rates, typically with those most affected being people who inject drugs, MSM and sex workers. And, although in many of these low prevalence countries the decline in new HIV infections appears to have stalled, the initial prevention responses were effective, and incidence rates declined rapidly until about 2000 or 2003.

One such picture of declining HIV incidence emerges in Malaysia (UNAIDS, 2014b), although the decline occurred later than in other South East Asia countries. In Malaysia, the national adult HIV prevalence is currently at 0.5 per cent, and the epidemic is concentrated in four most-at-risk or key populations (with prevalence >5 per cent): people who inject drugs; sex workers; MSM and transgender persons. Annual reports indicate a decline in numbers of HIV cases since 2002 (see Figure 1.2).

This decline appears to be the outcome of a number of prevention strategies. Harm-reduction initiatives – opioid substitution therapy (OST) and needles and syringe programmes (NSP) – were established in 2006 and are now located in a very large number of government health facilities. Prevention of sexual HIV transmission has also been pragmatically addressed using a number of strategies, including: sexually transmitted infection prevention services; outreach and peer education; behavioural-change communication and sexual

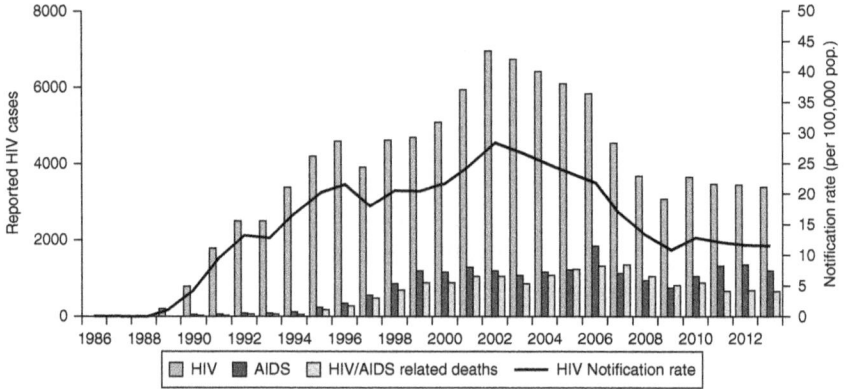

Figure 1.2 Malaysian reported HIV notification rate (1986–2013).

Source: Malaysian Country Report to UNAIDS, Malaysian Ministry of Health (2014, 13).

reproductive health education; encouragement of HIV testing; and counselling. The Malaysian Country Progress Report (2014) lists its best practices as harm reduction; enhancing prevention through partnership with Islamic bodies, including using a mosque as a place to provide methadone treatment to people who use drugs; and providing PMTCT.

Increasing HIV incidence

There is a third story to tell: some countries, for example, Pakistan and also countries that were part of the former Soviet Union – Belarus, Ukraine, Kazakhstan, Azerbaijan and Lithuania – are experiencing increases in HIV infections. These countries mostly have concentrated rather than generalised epidemics – primarily among people who inject drugs.

We take Ukraine as an example of increasing HIV incidence. In 2002 Ukraine documented 8,756 new infections, rising to almost 20,000 in 2009 and, in 2013, HIV incidence was recorded as 21,631. Reduction in the growth rate of this indicator was observed during 2006–2009: 16.8 per cent, 10.5 per cent, 7.6 per cent and 5.7 per cent respectively. It is recognised, however, that official data do not reflect the real scale of the HIV/AIDS epidemic in Ukraine, with questions about the reach of HIV testing and also about the extent to which HIV in migrants is identified and reported. Official notifications record 134,300 people living with HIV/AIDS and under medical observation in 2013 in comparison to national prevalence estimates of 238,000 HIV-infected people aged 15 and over living in Ukraine (UNAIDS, 2014b). The 2014 country report estimates that one-third of people who have tested positive for HIV as part of a prevalence study are not in contact with health services (either by not returning for their results or by making no contact with health services about their status). The difference between national prevalence estimates and prevalence figures based on notifications for 2013 suggests that a large proportion of HIV positive people in the Ukraine either do not know their status or are not accessing health services.

The number of HIV-positive people who inject drugs in Ukraine is of concern. Although the government supplies, and sanctions non-governmental organisations (NGOs) to supply, sterile needles and syringes to people who inject drugs through needle and syringe exchanges, the proportion of users reached by these programmes was estimated to be 63.9 per cent in 2013 (UNAIDS, 2014b). Furthermore young users report harassment by police, and many find it difficult to access HIV-prevention information.

Questions Raised

Although treatment is working, and more and more people living with HIV have access to ART, the picture with regard to prevention is complex, as signified by the differences between countries and the changes over time: HIV transmission rates are highly dependent on a range of social and cultural factors, as are HIV-prevention responses. The countries that have fared badly include those countries with generalised epidemics: that is, where HIV has mainly spread among the heterosexual population, as in southern Africa, and those countries experiencing increasing HIV incidence.

In an attempt to explain why, researchers have looked for answers in biology, ecology and the social and political sciences. For example, Stillwagon (2009) who, while acknowledging the importance of sexual behaviour, contends that the very high prevalence in southern Africa may be a function of the interaction of multiple biological characteristics of the host pathogen and environment. She argues that co-infection with other diseases such as malaria and schistosomiasis as well as long-term nutritional deficiencies make people far more vulnerable to HIV. Others have argued that iatrogenic transmission is part of the story, for example, Gisselquist, Potterat & Brody (2004). Mobility is also clearly implicated in the spread of HIV and, as noted by Thornton (2008), the mobility of workers in South Africa may explain in part the differential early HIV incidence between that country and Uganda.

It is highly likely that HIV transmission had been occurring in sub-Saharan Africa for at least 15 years before the virus was identified in 1983 and before a prevention response was developed: High prevalence makes effective prevention difficult. Furthermore, when the HIV response occurred it was understandably focused on treating the very large number of people living with

HIV and dying of AIDS. Although people recognised that HIV prevention was essential, there was and continues to be a tendency to see HIV prevention as part of the overall much-needed medical response and to provide prevention in the clinic. It is possible that this biomedical HIV-prevention response exacerbated an already very serious problem in the sense that, as discussed in Chapters 6 and 7, prevention works best if it arises from and is based in the community.

Those countries in which HIV is primarily transmitted via homosexual sex and via injecting have – with some notable exceptions – largely contained their epidemics within the populations in which these practices occur. Certainly different HIV transmission routes demand different prevention strategies. Countries with generalised epidemics will need different prevention strategies than those countries with concentrated epidemics. Generalised epidemics may be more difficult to contain than concentrated ones, and prevention strategies that are effective among heterosexuals may not work as well among gay and homosexually active men and vice versa. HIV transmission among people who inject drugs, too, will need very different strategies from those designed to prevent HIV sexual transmission.

We suggest that the sketches we have provided of different epidemics offer some ideas about how to account for some of the differential prevalence and incidence rates, but more detail is needed to inform prevention efforts. And as soon as we start to consider a deeper explanation, more questions arise. What accounts for the recent increases in a number of countries that initially were successful in reducing HIV transmission? Why have HIV infections been so difficult to reduce? What constitutes effective HIV prevention: Why have some countries fared better than others in reducing their HIV epidemic? This book offers a starting point for those trying to answer these questions in order to inform effective HIV prevention.

Reasons for the failure and success of HIV-prevention efforts

Given the differences in the patterning of HIV in the various regions and countries, and given the different modes of transmission, one HIV-prevention strategy will not suit all. Some possible reasons for poor HIV-prevention responses, noted by Friedman et al. (2006), include:

1. large-scale epidemics and related illness and death and their attendant social instability;
2. disruption caused by war, transitions, ecological disasters or economic failures;

3. government policies that ignore or defy evidence about 'what works';
4. the potential complacency of stable societies with low HIV prevalence;
5. biomedical advances and related opportunities as well as unintended costs.

As suggested above, with regard to the first of these, it is likely that in countries with high prevalence rates, treatment efforts are given priority over prevention. In Botswana, for instance, HIV prevention has been swamped by the need to treat people living with HIV. Although remarkable successes were achieved in ART coverage and PMTCT, the 2014 Botswana Country Progress Report documents the current challenges relating to prevention and notes the decreases in condom use and the continuing low levels of the basic HIV information (Botswana National AIDS Coordinating Agency, 2014, 18). A related issue concerns the funding of treatment and prevention responses to HIV. Botswana is one of many countries where there is real concern about the future as funds from the United States President's Emergency Plan for AIDS Relief (PEPFAR), the Bill & Melinda Gates Foundation and Merk are reduced (or withdrawn completely) – which leads to the second issue.

Large-scale disruptions may also lead to poor HIV-prevention responses. Wars and disruptions may interrupt social networks and undermine protective social norms, as Friedman & Reid (2002) demonstrate in South Africa. Economic downturns may lead to the mobility of people seeking employment and such mobility has contributed to high HIV-prevalence rates – at least in some countries such as South Africa (Thornton, 2008). In general, countries with poor economic outlooks will find it difficult to mount effective treatment and prevention responses. As Sam Friedman noted (personal communication), HIV infections among people who inject drugs increased in Greece when the needle and syringe programmes were closed as part of austerity measures.

Government policies, the third reason listed above, have clearly had an impact in those countries experiencing rapid increases among people who inject drugs, as in the Ukraine as discussed above. Although harm-reduction drug policies, including the provision of needle and syringe programmes, have now been accepted in the United States, as Drucker (2012) asks: How much could US policies have reduced the initial growth of the epidemic had harm reduction been instituted much earlier?

Illustrating the risks of optimism, it is noteworthy that HIV incidence figures pertaining to MSM in the income-rich world indicate the fragility of an ongoing strong HIV-prevention response. Since early in the twenty-first century most countries in Western Europe and North America as well as Australia and New Zealand have experienced increases in HIV incidence among MSM (Sullivan et al., 2014). It is entirely plausible that as the likelihood of death recedes in people's imaginations as the result of successful treatment in the form of ART, risk practices increase. As discussed in Chapter 3 and again in Chapter 6, the evidence supports this hypothesis – at least with reference to gay communities in low prevalence, income-rich parts of the world.

And finally, there is some evidence – as discussed in Chapter 7, that recent increases in HIV in many countries may be related to biomedical advances in the form of pre-exposure prophylaxis (PrEP) and TasP – or at least the unintended consequences of the rhetoric surrounding these advances. And, although many in biomedicine believe that 'test and treat', in the context of widespread testing and early uptake of and adherence to treatment, will reduce HIV transmission, consideration of some of the distinct patterns in HIV epidemics across the world casts doubt on claims about the universal promise of ART, in the form of TasP, as an effective means of prevention. Although there is little if any doubt with regard to the efficacy of TasP, the accumulating 'real world' data tell a different, more complex, story about the *effectiveness* of TasP.

Prevention and Treatment

Notwithstanding the overall declines in HIV incidence, there is a growing unease that prevention has stalled – in part because its impact is so uneven and because a proportion of people continue to seroconvert. Many biomedical scientists have claimed that HIV prevention efforts have been having less of an impact than earlier (for example, Potts et al., 2008). Some, such as Maggiolo & Leone (2010), have argued that 'disappointing' biomedical interventions and 'unsatisfactory results' of interventions that rely on behaviour change account for the failure. Still others in public health, such as Granich et al. (2013), have argued that an 'AIDS-free generation' is both scientifically sound and practically feasible and have pinned their hopes on the relatively new biomedical strategies based on treatment (ART) for, and as, prevention.

Coupled with the unease about the uneven outcomes of prevention, the success of treatment has led to a remedicalising of HIV prevention efforts. It is our claim that one of the factors related to this recent stalling of prevention has been the lack of attention in many countries to the social aspects of what is a very social disease, and that the more recent remedicalisation of HIV prevention, with its whole-hearted embrace of the biomedical paradigm and the turn to 'prevention in the clinic', has exacerbated the problem. While HIV prevention has always been seen by many in biomedicine as a 'medical' issue, the medicalisation of HIV prevention has intensified since the effectiveness of using ART for the prevention of

HIV from mother to child programmes was demonstrated in the late 1990s. Globally, ART is now successfully used to reduce the transmission of HIV from an HIV-infected mother to her child during pregnancy, labour, delivery and breastfeeding, although there are still gaps in delivery and access in some countries (WHO, 2014). The search for biomedical solutions in the form of pre- and post-exposure prophylaxis also began in the late 1990s, and the most recent move has been to advocate placing all those with HIV on treatment as soon as possible after they are infected in order to reduce ongoing transmission.

Many in public health now speak of the 'prevention and treatment continuum', but the insistence that prevention and treatment are on some sort of linear continuum or, worse, the collapsing of one into the other is misleading – at least until an effective prophylactic vaccine is developed. The practice of ingesting drugs to *treat* infectious diseases is a common one, and one that most people understand. Although there are examples where drug ingestion *prevents* or reduces the likelihood of diseases such as malaria, the ongoing daily ingestion of prophylactic drugs to prevent infectious diseases is not common. Given the global scale of HIV, such a response may prove difficult to implement as well as extremely costly.

Beyond accounting for failure, it is vital to understand what produces successful prevention strategies. In the countries that have witnessed a sustained HIV prevention response – those countries in Western Europe and North America, Asia and the Pacific and Latin America – there is evidence of community engagement and involvement in prevention. Similarly, the early successful response in Uganda was underpinned by a level of public discussion, debate and involvement that appears not to have been sustained. As mentioned, and as discussed in Chapters 2, 3 and 6, in many high-income countries not only were alliances struck with gay, bisexual and other men who have sex with men, sex workers, and people who inject drugs and, in the case of Uganda, with village elders, but collaborations were also established with progressive religious organisations – as in Brazil and Malaysia – and with labour unions, women's health and feminist organisations, youth groups and the emerging Black movement in Brazil. Perhaps the most important lesson from these responses to the HIV epidemic has been their circumvention of individualistic prevention strategies and their focus on working with communities to change their social worlds.

These early successful HIV prevention responses were essentially social in the sense that, to a greater or lesser extent, in each country prevention strategies were built with the populations most at risk 'at the table', and collaborations were forged with a range of cultural institutions. Indeed, many of the HIV-prevention strategies emerged from communities before public health endorsed them: for example, condom use. While other strategies, such as those that rely on ART and male circumcision, were introduced via bio-medicine. The *efficacy* of the range of HIV-prevention strategies varies, and it is likely that some, if not all, have played a role and will continue to play a role in reducing HIV infection. The degree to which they are *effective* in the real world is a function of whether the strategies are taken up and their use embraced and sustained over time by people – both those at risk of HIV infec-tion and those at risk of transmitting HIV. That is, their effectiveness hinges on whether they are built into people's everyday social practices. Effectiveness also depends on whether governments and their various arms, such as their educational and public health departments, invest in informing, promoting and making the technologies easily available and affordable, be they condoms, sterile needles and syringes, or ART in its various forms.

The picture is complex: the declines in incidence are not strong enough and in many countries have not been sustained. Are the prevention strategies we have available good enough? Are they being deployed and taken up in ways that maximise their effectiveness? Are they sustainable? Nothing has produced more debate in the field of HIV prevention than the question of the effective-ness of various HIV-prevention strategies.

While we agree that prevention has stalled, our argument is that it has stalled because the social worlds in which HIV is transmitted have been overlooked and, in Fassin's terms, the social has been rendered practically inexpressible. This has happened as the emphasis on biomedical approaches to prevention has become greater and greater, as we show in Chapter 4. Unless an effective vaccine is produced, there is no 'magic bullet'. Prevention responses of the past twenty-five or so years have taught us a great deal, principally that what works and what will work to reduce HIV incidence is contingent. The social transformation required to support changes in people's practices may not hap-pen in a linear fashion, and it takes time.

Effective HIV prevention is complex: what works 'here' may not work 'there', what worked 'then' may not work 'now' or in the 'future', and what worked for 'us' may not work for 'them'. Answers to why some HIV-prevention strategies have worked better than others and some countries have fared bet-ter than others in containing and reducing their epidemics are what this book attempts to provide. This book shows that effective prevention is to be found in the interaction between social structures and the people who transform or reproduce them – that is, in the social relations *between* people and how these social relations are brought into play with regard to these intimate practices of sex and drug injection so that they are, or can be, made safer with regard to HIV transmission.

We begin to provide answers to 'what works' and 'why' in the next two chapters, where we detail the prevention responses of two very different countries, Uganda and Australia, both of which demonstrate in very different ways – at least initially – the success of a genuine community response and the development of a 'social vaccine'.

Chapter 2

'OWNING' UGANDA

We start our analysis of global HIV prevention by considering two moments in the Ugandan epidemic, an epidemic that has already come under intense scrutiny: moment one, between 2000 and 2014 and moment two, the late 1980s to 1990s. Despite sustained calls by the Joint United Nations Programme on HIV/AIDS (UNAIDS) to 'know your epidemic' (Wilson & Halperin, 2008; UNAIDS, 2014c) – to understand its nuances and specificities – much of the extensive interrogation of Uganda's epidemic to date has clouded an understanding of shifts in HIV transmission and prevention. Here we analyse reports and accounts of Ugandan prevention efforts, distinguishing between the social practices Ugandans developed to respond to HIV and the retrospective identification of 'individual behaviours' put forward as instances of 'Abstinence, B[eing] Faithful, [Using] Condoms' (ABC).

Uganda is about the same geographic size as the United Kingdom, with a population of nearly 36 million people and an HIV prevalence in adults of currently 7.3 per cent (although overall prevalence is higher in urban populations, prevalence is rising in rural populations) (Uganda AIDS Commission, 2014). Relative to some other African countries, 7.2 per cent may not seem high (for example, Swaziland or Botswana), however an estimated 1.6 million Ugandans (children and adults under 50) are living with HIV (Uganda AIDS Commission, 2014). Of more concern, HIV incidence has risen in recent years, with no significant decline – new infections in adults in 2011 were 134,634, in 2012 were 139,178 and in 2013 were 131,279 (Uganda AIDS Commission, 2014).

Moment One: 2000–2014

Prevalence has also risen with the upturn located around 2003–2004 (Green & Ruark, 2011), an estimate confirmed by recent biannual country reports

(Uganda AIDS Commission, 2012) documenting the HIV prevalence among antenatal clinic (ANC) attendees (see Figure 2.1).

This increase in HIV prevalence is due not only to the impact of treatment, but also to an increase in HIV incidence. UNAIDS figures show a small but steady rise in HIV incidence from the early 2000s to 2009 (see Figure 2.2).

The HIV incidence figures indicate a 16.4 per cent rise in adult incidence between the reporting periods 2007–2008 and 2009–2010 (Uganda AIDS Commission, 2012). The Uganda AIDS Commission explains that '[a]ccording to the Mode of Transmission study carried out in 2008, it was found that most of the new infections are in the context of stable long term partnerships' (2012, 11). The 2013 Country Progress Report (Uganda AIDS Commission 2014, 5) also considers what might be contributing to HIV incidence and on the basis of modelling estimates that 43 per cent of new infections in adults are occurring in 'mutually monogamous heterosexual relationships;

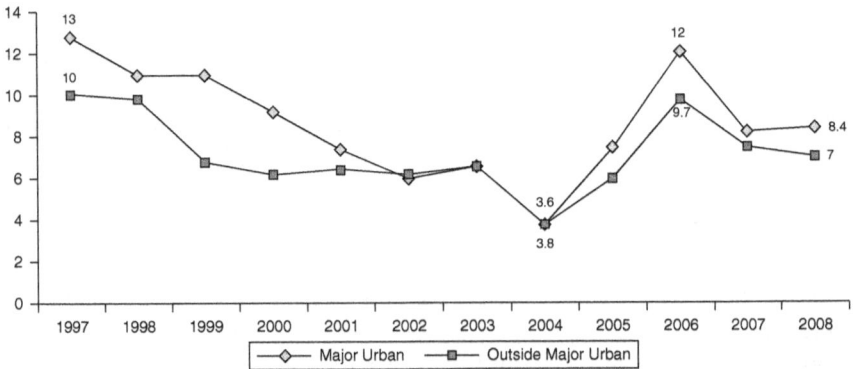

Figure 2.1 Median HIV prevalence of ANC attendees from major towns and outside (1997–2008).

Source: Ugandan Aids Commission, Progress Report (2012, 7).

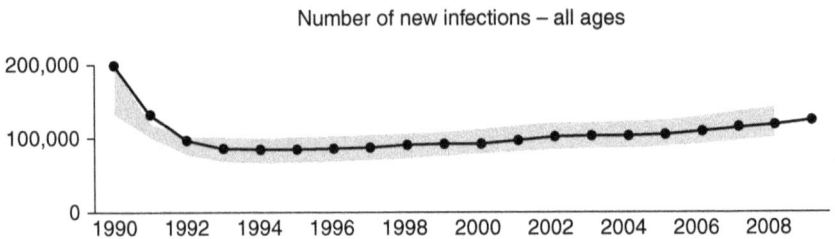

Figure 2.2 UNAIDS country information, Uganda.

Source: http://www.unaids.org/en/regionscountries/countries/uganda/ (accessed September 18, 2013).

while another 46 per cent were among persons in multiple sexual unions'. Ugandan prevention of mother-to-child transmission (PMTCT) coverage has expanded, and the estimated HIV prevalence in infants born to HIV positive women has fallen (from 19.4% to 7.4% between 2007–2008 and 2010–2011). Incidence in infants was not contributing to the country's overall increase, but new infections in adults were (Uganda AIDS Commission, 2012).

Why has incidence risen? Given that in earlier years the Ugandan epidemic has been subjected to so much analysis, we might expect the components of an answer to lie in the ideas circulating about Uganda's former success in HIV prevention, in the form of understandings of the dynamics of HIV prevention and transmission in Uganda and the way these dynamics have changed. So, we turn to the past.

Moment Two: The Late 1980s–1990s

There is widespread recognition of Uganda's HIV-prevention 'success' in the late 1980s and early 1990s. Figure 2.2 (above) from UNAIDS shows a decline in HIV incidence from 1990 to 1995, but there is much to indicate that it extends back to the late 1980s. The 1993–1994 Ugandan HIV prevalence figures showed a sharp decline (Asiimwe-Okirer et al., 1995; Stoneburner et al., 1996). Low-Beer and Stoneburner (2004) estimated that the decline in HIV prevalence was preceded by a decline in incidence in the late 1980s or early 1990s. Accurate incidence figures are often hard to collect and one (widely accepted) proxy gauge is prevalence in pregnant women: Low-Beer & Stoneburner (2004) identified a drop in national figures from 21.1 per cent to 6 per cent in the decade between 1991 and 2000. The fact that the declines in younger women (a closer gauge of incidence) were more marked (see Figure 2.3) further indicates the validity of this proxy measure of incidence. Between 1991 and 2002, HIV prevalence in male army recruits (aged 21 years) also declined from 18 per cent to below 4 per cent (Low-Beer & Stoneburner, 2004).[1]

Although the decline in prevalence has been contested as a meaningful indicator of decline in incidence, the counter explanations do not hold up. For example, fertility biases (for example, the idea that over time HIV positive women are less likely to become pregnant and therefore less likely to be present in antenatal surveillance) do not explain the same declining trend in young male recruits, and mortality does not explain the sharp declines in younger people (Asiimwe-Okiror et al., 1997; UNAIDS, 1999; Low-Beer & Stone-burner, 2004). Ugandans had to be doing something to make this turnaround in their epidemic. There is a clear account of what Ugandans did in the years preceding the decline in incidence. They embraced the problem of HIV and openly discussed and acted on ways to reduce transmission, including delaying

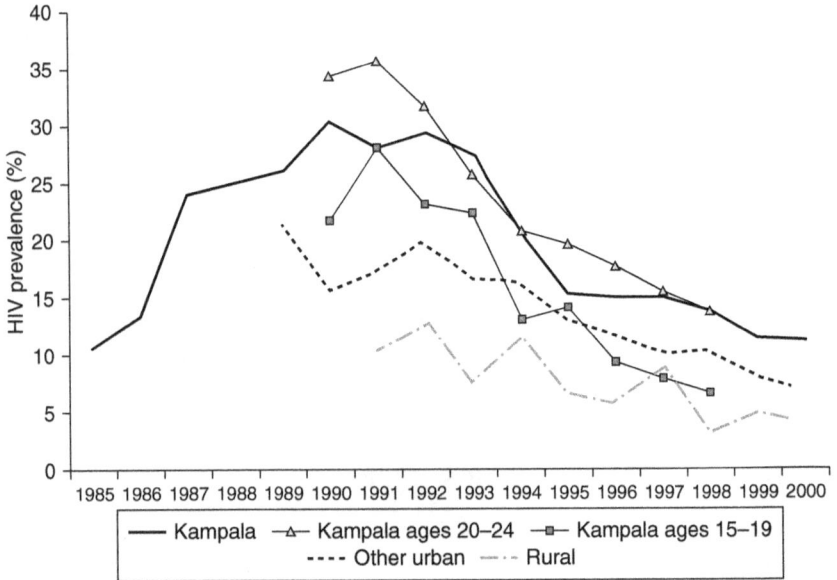

Figure 2.3 HIV prevalence rates (%) in pregnant women surveyed at antenatal sentinel surveillance sites in Uganda in urban Kampala, other urban sentinel sites, and rural sites (1985–2001).

Source: Stoneburner, R. & Low-Beer, D. (2004). Population-level HIV declines and behavioural risk avoidance in Uganda. *Science*, 304, 714–718. Reprinted with permission from AAAS.

sexual initiation; reducing the number of their sexual partners; and using condoms. Their engagement with HIV became part of the social fabric, developing what Low-Beer & Stoneburner (2004) have described as a 'social vaccine' with 75 per cent effectiveness.

The social vaccine: Social relations/ social norms/social practice

The explanation for what Ugandans did hinges on examining changes in social relations – not only sexual relations between partners, but the way that HIV materialised in social relations of all kinds. One clear indication of this comes from Low-Beer & Stoneburner's comparison of Ugandan Demographic and Health Survey (DHS) data (1989 and 1995) with other African countries with generalised epidemics. Ugandans' 'knowledge' of HIV did not markedly differ from other countries. What did distinguish Ugandans was that in 1995, when questioned about how people heard and communicated about HIV, Ugandans alone reported the importance of personal relationships with friends and relatives as source of information about HIV, as compared with public media (including radio, TV, pamphlets, but also churches and community centres). The existence of these horizontal (as opposed to vertical, top-down) communication networks about HIV suggests that *HIV had taken root in everyday social relations in Uganda* (Low-Beer & Stoneburner, 2003; 2004). In addition most Ugandans reported personally knowing someone with AIDS (91.5% of men and 86.4% of women) – indicating a connection to HIV unlike those reported in other African countries – including those with similarly large epidemics.[2] On the basis of their analysis of these data, Low-Beer & Stoneburner argue that Ugandans integrated HIV into social relations via 'a *community communication* process [...] different from individual knowledge, or even communication between partners' (2004, 179), a development they characterise as a 'social vaccine'.

Both the patterning of Uganda's epidemic and the potency of their 'social vaccine' are specific to time and place. Thornton's (2008) ethnographic comparison of Ugandans and South Africans identifies the role of political history in shaping very different kinds of sexual networks in Uganda and South Africa, with different possibilities for HIV transmission. Under apartheid, South Africa became a country where migration for work became the norm, meaning much of the population was mobile and living in communities comprised of different ethnicities and backgrounds. Sexual networks covered large distances, and each 'node' of connection potentially opened out into many more clusters. In contrast, Ugandans' systems of land tenure were never completely broken, and populations there were much more ethnically integrated than were populations in South Africa. Thornton argues that Ugandan sexual networks were also more stable and relatively isolated. This means that the consequences of any changes Ugandans made in their sexual practices were more likely to readily manifest as declines in HIV incidence.

The potency of Uganda's 'social vaccine' also needs to be understood, as it connects to political shifts. HIV was widely and publicly discussed in Uganda in the early and mid-1980s, *before* Musevini came to power in January 1986. Newspaper coverage in the 1980s gives some indications of the intense public discussion and debates Ugandans were having about a disease variously known as SIRIIMU, slim, SILIIMU or SSILIMU (Thornton, 2008). Thornton argues that open discussions at a community level resulted in 'Ugandans accept[ing] the reality of the disease' (2008, 115). The Ugandan women's movement quickly took up HIV as a central concern, and pressured the new government to change rape, divorce and property rights legislation at the same time as encouraging people to educate girls (Ankrah, 1992; Epstein, 2007). Local support organisations were established to care for people with HIV including, in 1987, The AIDS Support Organization (TASO), which

established a system of home-based care and actively countered stigma, discrimination and misinformation about transmission (Ankrah, 1992; Epstein,
2007). Through this public discussion and action, Ugandans came to largely
recognise HIV as *their* problem, rather than as an external problem visited
upon them. And although, as Thornton (2008) noted, early Ugandan newspaper coverage included suggestions that HIV was being brought to the
country by foreigners, discussion of HIV as an external problem waned as
understanding of HIV grew. Accepting the reality of HIV was not a straightforward case of Ugandan people 'acquiring knowledge', but it involved close
attention to and debate over the details of their own epidemic which, in turn,
by the end of the 1980s led to widespread understanding of HIV as heterosexually transmitted.

Explanations of Uganda's success commonly and too readily foreground
Museveni's 'good political leadership' as *leading* to changes in sexual practice
and thus essentially holding to a top-down account of social change. However,
social research that attends to what *Ugandans were doing* suggests that 'the [com-
munity] response preceded and exceeded HIV interventions. Ugandans managed their epidemic, took credit for success, and national and international
policy provided support and built on the people's response, rather than the
other way around. HIV policy was developed and prevention started in the vil-
lages, and political and public health interventions built on this' (Low-Beer &
Stoneburner, 2004, 182). The mechanism that enabled this collective response
to HIV was not a particular message or health-promotion intervention (Allen
& Heald, 2004; Allen, 2006; Swidler, 2009). Rather, social mobilisation triggered shifts in the social norms shaping the meaning of sexual relationships
and sexual practice.

Public health: Harnessing and fuelling the social vaccine

Museveni's interest in addressing HIV was reportedly triggered by a call from
Fidel Castro in 1986 to inform him that more than 25 per cent of the Ugandan military personnel sent to Cuba for training had tested HIV positive. His
new government quickly harnessed, supported and facilitated community
initiatives when it came to power at the end of the civil war following Idi
Amin's rule. In October 1986, just months after Museveni came to power,
the new minister of health, Batwala, implemented a public-information campaign explicitly linking HIV prevention to national reconstruction. Early
national HIV-prevention campaigns largely targeting men (Zero Grazing/
Love Carefully) were established (billboards, media messages, mobile HIV
vans with messages) soon after in 1987. Also in 1987 teachers were trained to

do comprehensive HIV education in schools (Human Rights Watch, 2005). Government supported condom provision began in 1989.

Certainly, the Ugandan response to HIV entailed public health messages to give people information and knowledge. However, we need to move beyond discussing the content of messages and their mode of delivery to how people engage with these messages and, more generally, reach an understanding of their role in social change. Responding to HIV was given a particular meaning: the new government approached tackling HIV as a means to promote civil engagement. HIV prevention was framed as part of rebuilding the nation, a very public and collective concern (Low-Beer & Stoneburner, 2004; Allen, 2006). In this way not just individual choices, but social norms of sexual practice were specifically linked to the political future of the nation. The mechanism for making this connection was a decentralised response, officially initiated in 1988. This response took shape in the form of local 'Resistance Councils', named as such because this level of local government evolved from regional rebel-support structures in areas controlled by Museveni-aligned forces before he came to power (they were renamed local councils in the mid-1990s). These Resistance Councils involved medical staff, community leaders and the members of local and international non-governmental organisations (NGOs) who together took responsibility for local HIV-prevention efforts (Ankrah, 1992). Members of the councils visited households to inform people about HIV and facilitated community meetings at which possible responses to HIV were discussed and debated. Thus the government agenda of linking HIV to national reconstruction by rebuilding civil society was manifest in the architecture of the response to HIV. This institutional approach harnessed, supported and fuelled ongoing local level public discussions about HIV, and HIV incidence rapidly declined.

A 'Ugandan' public health

Uganda was remarkably successful in garnering international funding for HIV in ways that it had not previously managed for broader development (Parkhurst, 2005). The Ugandan public health response has entailed a wide array of international actors. From the outset in 1987 the World Health Organization (WHO) funding supported the establishment of the National Committee for the Prevention of AIDS together with the Ministry of Health AIDS Control Program (ACP) with responsibility for HIV prevention; surveillance; blood screening and testing; and training of medical personnel and public leaders (Ankrah, 1992; Parkhurst, 2005). WHO had senior staff on the ACP from its inception and the first national action plan (1987) charged WHO with guiding HIV prevention (Parkhurst, 2005). Multiple international agencies, local hospitals and NGOs were involved, including the Red Cross, World Vision, Save the Children Fund, UNICEF, USAID and the World Bank (Ankrah, 1992). Donor funding, administered by a WHO 'trust fund', came from the United Kingdom, Sweden, United States, Denmark, Norway and Italy in addition to bilateral funding (Parkhurst, 2005). Two things are noteworthy about this international involvement. First, although external advice and funding *could have* effectively delegitimised the government, the Ugandan government carved out a role for itself that went beyond harnessing international expertise to inform the development of the national strategy. This role included overseeing and integrating multiple and diverse HIV-prevention approaches into the national response (Parkhurst, 2005). The new government was strengthened by international involvement in HIV. Second, in Museveni's early years, the government did not dictate the best means of HIV prevention to local Resistance Councils or to international actors involved: the response was multiple and diverse and is best characterised as a massive social experiment.

The 'end product' of the social vaccine: Changes in sexual practice

Social mobilisation supported by multiple local and national public health responses and agencies brought about changes in Ugandans' sexual practices. These changes have been largely discussed as 'individual behaviour changes' and documented by Green & Ruark (2011, 169):

1. A sharp decline between 1989 and 1995 in premarital sex on the part of young people (15–24 years), in men from 60 per cent to 23 per cent and in women from 53 per cent to 16 per cent;
2. Declines between 1989 and 1995 in 'high risk' sex ('high risk' here as it is being used to mean *any* sex between people who are not married or cohabitating irrespective of condom use or negotiations grounded in knowledge of HIV status); in adult men from 41 per cent to 21 per cent, and in adult women, from 23 per cent to 9 per cent;
3. Declines in the number of men reporting three or more non-regular partners from 15 per cent (in the past year, 1989) to 3 per cent (in the past six months, 1995);
4. Increases between 1989 and 1995 in the rates of people reporting 'ever' having used a condom from 15 per cent to 30 per cent of men and 7 per cent to 20 per cent of women. Low-Beer & Stoneburner (2004) note that in the 1995 DHS, 12.5 per cent of men (20 per cent of unmarried and 8 per cent of married) reported having adopted condoms as a HIV-prevention strategy, and 2.9 per cent of women.

With regard to condom use, Green & Ruark (2011) note that 'ever' having used a condom is not a particularly useful indicator of an effective HIV-prevention strategy and are wary of attributing the observed changes in HIV transmission to the use of condoms. Furthermore, Low-Beer & Stoneburner (2004) note that levels of condom use on the part of Ugandans do not stand out as very different from countries where there were no declines in prevalence in this period and concur that the early Ugandan success cannot be *largely* attributed to condom use. The decline does seem to be connected to a reduction in the number of partners on the part of those who were sexually active, and delaying sexual debut. However while we agree that 'ever using condoms' is not a very useful measure and measures of 'how often' and 'with whom' condoms are used are needed, there were large increases as demonstrated by this restricted measure of condom use between 1989 and 1995. Furthermore, as we show later, the decrease in condom use associated with the later increase in HIV incidence is indicative that condoms played some part in the early decline.

In this account of the changes in social practice – typically discussed as 'behaviour changes' – we can see connections to the three components of an approach to HIV prevention named and proliferated a decade *after* Uganda's success: 'Abstinence, Be faithful, use Condoms' or, ABC. Although ABC *could* mean engaging people simultaneously with three different possible modes of HIV prevention, in effect its US proponents worked on the basis of promoting 'Abstinence for unmarried youth, Being faithful for married couples, and Condom use for "those who are infected or who are unable to avoid high-risk behaviours (such as discordant couples)"' (PEPFAR, 2004, cited in Human Rights Watch, 2005, 22).

International discussion of Uganda was quickly colonised and constrained by the idea that HIV prevention could be reduced to a retrospective assessment of ABC (Green et al., 2006; Gray et al., 2006; Singh et al., 2004; Slutkin et al., 2006). Yet '[v]eteran AIDS educators in Uganda had never heard of "ABC" until the United States branded Uganda's success with this alphabetical sound-bite' (Human Rights Watch, 2005, 6). This mismatch between what HIV educators understood they themselves to be doing during the early turnaround in Uganda's epidemic, and retrospective discussion by researchers, evidences the problem of discussing HIV prevention as behaviour change devoid of any analysis of the history, context and meanings that people ascribe to their social practices (Seeley, 2015). Such discussions offer glimpses of the social change involved – the changes in sexual practice – but give little insight into the mechanisms of social change that enabled Ugandans to engage with HIV, to openly discuss it, to see it as something they needed to devise responses to and then to act.

What Happened in Between These Two Moments in Uganda's Epidemic?

International attention to Ugandan's HIV-prevention success clouded the importance of the role that open public discussion of HIV played in changes to social practice. This was not a coincidence. Initially, any attention at all was very slow to develop. Early international recognition of the declines in incidence and prevalence was marked by disbelief on the part of international researchers (although not by most Ugandan researchers or by Low-Beer & Stoneburner) and by attempts to explain away successful HIV prevention by attributing the figures to mortality or fertility biases in sentinel surveillance data.

The debate about 'what worked' revolved around the problem of evidence in public health with many demanding evidence of the type afforded by randomised controlled trials (RCTs) rather than the available descriptive evidence. In Uganda, the evidence connecting population-wide epidemiological data to prevention strategies and approaches developed over time by a loose assemblage of people, government and the wide array of non-governmental and international actors is extremely complex and not based on RCTs (Kippax, 2003; Parkhurst, 2008) and many did not accept it. The ground was fertile for confusion and ongoing debate. However, this complexity does not explain the fact that the debate did not really build until the 2000s – nearly a decade after the success was first noticed (Low-Beer & Stoneburner, 2004). At this point the field of global HIV prevention was rapidly opening up to a new array of powerful actors, in particular the US President's Emergency Plan for AIDS Relief (PEPFAR), with questionable investments in characterising 'successful HIV prevention' as A and B, not C (Cohen & Tate, 2006).

PEPFAR needed evidence for the effectiveness of promoting abstinence (A) for unmarried people and fidelity (B) for married people (Human Rights Watch, 2005). Abstinence-only programmes had been tried and tested in the United States and shown to fail (Cohen, Schleifer & Tate, 2005); and Uganda's government promised to provide the evidence required – and not only through its place in the international debate about Ugandan incidence figures, but in person. Lady Janet Museveni's 2003 address to the US Congress played an important role in the United States in legitimising PEPFAR's notion of AB HIV prevention. She claimed that Uganda's adoption of AB explained the downturn in their epidemic. As Cooper (2015, 69) notes, 'Her visit reportedly secured the $1 billion earmarked for abstinence and faithfulness in the final bill and earned her the enduring gratitude of American Evangelicals. It also ensured that Uganda would become one of the largest single recipients of PEPFAR funding'.[3] Thus while debates over Uganda's success were conducted along the lines of 'evidence' and how best to understand it, what fuelled the debates was the unrolling of a US-formulated faith-based ideological approach to HIV prevention (Bass, 2005). This meant that retrospective examination of the Ugandan epidemic was animated by efforts to find evidence of the effectiveness of A and B when these programmes were being pushed across the globe by PEPFAR.[4]

The discussion of Ugandan HIV responses can be seen as an extension of the 1990s US 'culture wars' – divisive public debates over so called 'hot-button' issues like abortion, drug use, homosexuality and gun control (Green, Halperin, Nantulya & Hogle, 2006). The culture wars afforded particular messianic versions of Christianity increasing power not only to shape national politics in the United States but also, through international aid such as PEPFAR, to shape global health (Cooper, 2015). The upshot was that, although many eyes were turned to Uganda, few were actually interrogating the details of what Ugandans had done, and few were looking at what was happening in the present: first, incidence stopped declining, and then it increased. Political and public health discussion of Uganda's success, which was framed in terms of A and B, preceded rising HIV incidence and, more recently, a Ugandan version of the culture wars resulted in the passing of the Uganda Anti-Homosexuality Act in February 2014, punishing homosexuality in the country with life imprisonment (life imprisonment having replaced the death sentence that was proposed and debated throughout 2013). In August 2014, the Anti-Homosexuality Act was overturned by the Constitutional Court and was followed by a 'gay pride' rally.

The debate over evidence and the relative roles of A, B and C is framed, discussed and pushed as a matter of 'individual behaviours' that are potentially generalisable and universalisable, with the result that the terrain of HIV prevention is cast as static and unchanging. Such a static picture means that some analysts lament the past: consider Green & Ruark's (2011) argument that increases in new infections have followed Ugandans' turning away from some of their late 1980s and early 1990s behaviour changes (that is, less sex outside of monogamous partnerships, less premarital sex) and towards condoms and other supposedly 'non-Ugandan' solutions that they see as clouding and confusing HIV prevention today. Such arguments fail to grasp that what has worked in the past did so because it addressed the way that HIV was manifest and understood in the past, and that what will work today will do so because it engages with the manifestation of HIV today. Furthermore, it is not true to assert that the promotion of condoms in Uganda is disrupting HIV prevention, as we show below.

What happened to Uganda's social vaccine? Going back to the country's initial success, the Ugandan response was distinguished by open public discussion about living with, dying from, and preventing HIV and, to some degree, about sex – at least as framed by HIV. This public discussion enabled changes in the norms regulating sexual practice. Maintaining discussion as the epidemic changes is needed to enable people to continue to identify the familiar as well as the newly manifested challenge of HIV prevention and to develop changes to social practice. However, today, there are indications that Ugandans are less open to publicly discussing HIV. When asked in 2006 if they would advise a family member who tested positive to keep their status secret (Uganda Bureau of Statistics, 2007, 2012), 53 per cent of women and 62 per cent of men did not agree with secrecy (that is, tending towards openness); but in 2011 these figures were lower, at 39.8 per cent and 54.3 per cent, respectively. This suggests that HIV status became *more* private between 2006 and 2011. A recent re-analysis of these data together with data collected from HIV participants in a treatments study (2007–2012) concludes that '[i]nternalised stigma has increased over time among PLHIV [People Living with HIV/AIDS] in the setting of worsening anticipated stigma in the general population' (Chan et al., 2015, 83). There are also indications that the idea of open discussion with young people about sex and condoms is more fraught for Ugandan women today than a decade ago: asked if 12–14 year olds should be taught about condoms in school, 25.3 per cent of women thought not in 2000–2001,[5] but in 2011 36.5 per cent of women did not support the idea (Uganda Bureau of Statistics, 2001, 2012). Contemporary research, discussed below, suggests that although many young people in rural areas are flouting expectations of virginity until marriage, the possibilities for any kind of collective discussion of what they are doing are highly constrained. The recent landscape of HIV prevention appears to be silencing public discussion of many aspects of HIV.

The promotion of abstinence and fidelity and the sidelining of condoms (PEPFAR)

Ugandans' 'horizontal' public discussion of HIV between family and friends was replaced over time by vertical and 'top-down' information from government, churches, schools and other authorities. The 'social vaccine', which had been so effective, was undermined, and the social practices that had enabled Ugandans to reduce HIV transmission – delaying sexual initiation, reducing the number of sexual partners and condom use – were repackaged as AB and not C, or only C in circumstances defined as sex outside a cohabiting relationship, which is nonsensical given, as mentioned, so many new infections – 43 per cent – are attributable to sex in long-term, mutually monogamous relationships.

PEPFAR funding shaped the terrain of HIV prevention by exempting faith-based organisations from including materials or information that they found morally objectionable and legislating that at least one-third of prevention funds be spent on abstinence-only programmes (PEPFAR Watch, http://www.pepfarwatch.org/). In the 2008 reauthorisation of funding this was changed so that if more than 50 per cent of prevention funds were spent on 'non-abstinence' strategies, a report was required by Congress explaining why. The 2003 legislation also dictated that PEPFAR funding was to be restricted to organisations that publicly pledged an anti–sex-work position: legislation that was deemed unconstitutional by the US Supreme Court in June 2013 on the basis that that it inhibited the free speech of recipient agencies, although the implications of this ruling have yet to unfold. Also, PEPFAR does not fund the proven prevention strategy of clean needle and syringe provision.

Uganda played an important role in PEPFAR experimentation and solidification well before Lady Museveni's appearance before the US Congress. The previous year, in 2002, Uganda availed itself of US funding from the Presidential Initiative on AIDS Strategy for Communication to Youth (PIASCY) and developed a school-based HIV-prevention programme. Although the messages now taught in schools are predominantly about abstinence, this initially was not the case, and the first draft of the national school-based HIV-prevention education included information about condoms and safe sex for young people. In 2003, however, with the influence of evangelical groups, references to condoms were removed in favour of a new pro-abstinence chapter on 'ethics and morals' (Cohen & Tate, 2006; Human Rights Watch, 2005). The programme entails didactically taught messages and spectacular events such as rallies to access youth outside of school – vertical approaches to communication that potentially counter the horizontal modes of communication that distinguished the Ugandan social vaccine in the early years. A critical analysis of current Ugandan sex-education policies, including PIASCY (Iyer & Aggleton, 2014), identified the different strategies for protecting youth extending across educational levels: primary abstinence from sex was to be promoted to students in primary and secondary educational institutions, while knowledge, skills and values that promote faithfulness and condom-use education were to be delayed until tertiary education. The analysis also revealed that the language used in PIASCY was overtly religious. In PIASCY '[i]t is asserted that in the African context, and with all religious convictions and practices in Uganda, sex outside of marriage is not approved' (2014, 436) and that virginity is a key Ugandan value.

Rijsdijk et al. (2013) found major discrepancies between the political and economic contexts of young people's lives and the norms and values that current sex education attempts to instil in students in educational institutions. Not only are messages promoting abstinence and delaying sexual initiation being flouted by many young people, they are not being subjected to collective scrutiny or discussion. Bell's research (Bell, 2011; Bell & Aggleton, 2012) examines the social context in which young people conduct their sexual relationships prior to marriage in three rural Ugandan regions. Increasingly, marriage for girls is being delayed, partly so that they can avail themselves of educational opportunities.[6] Girls are 'protected' from sexual activity by keeping them busy at home when not at school – a practice that isolates them and minimises their opportunities to connect with trusted adults and any existing services where they could discuss their sexual lives. For boys and young men, although the punitive Ugandan defilement law for sex with a woman under 18 years is not formally exercised (death or up to 18-year prison sentences), Bell (2011) identified local imprisonment, the payment of fines to the girls' parents and impoverishment as punishments. These constraints mean, Bell argues, that while young people often exercise 'subtle agency' in the sense that they still find ways to have sex and sexual relationships, without collective acknowledgement and discussion, these many acts of transgression do not build into any form of public challenge to, or reworking of, the social norms and expectations in place (2011, 294). In contrast to the public discussion of the late 1980s to early 1990s (the social vaccine), sex for young people is marked by secrecy.

Beyond school-based education, the Ugandan AIDS Commission, together with the Young Empowered and Healthy (YEAH) campaign, developed with international funding a series of radio shows, events and other communication channels targeting young people, 15–24 years old, to try to change what PEPFAR saw as problematic social norms. Between 2005 and 2008 these efforts focused on reducing transactional sex and challenging gender norms, but avoided broader discussions about safe sex beyond marriage, condom use or HIV transmission between monogamous couples. The messages were about abstinence, delaying sex, fidelity and acting respectfully toward oneself and others. YEAH was not the first media campaign specifically targeting young people; there had been others, most notably *Straight Talk*. Established in newspaper insert format in 1993 (initially funded by UNICEF), *Straight Talk* grew into a monthly newspaper produced in seven different languages, as well as local radio programmes broadcast in 11 languages by 2006. This initiative was an attempt to act on the findings of Grunseit & Kippax's (1993) review of sex education for WHO's Global Programme on AIDS, which identified that efforts to increase the age of sexual initiation were best supported by messages about delaying sex rather than abstinence, and that effective education involves conveying negotiation skills, not just facts. *Straight Talk* began by communicating and encouraging discussion of a range of HIV-prevention strategies to adolescents. However, following the 2004 introduction of ABC,

Straight Talk found it 'had to be self-conscious about what it was writing' (Adamchack et al., 2007, 6). Furthermore, a review of its impact conducted in 2005–2006 identified that, while nearly 70 per cent of the respondents (aged 10–18 years, mean age 14.5 years, 12% of whom had had sex) said that their action involved adopting abstinence as a consequence of reading *Straight Talk*, fewer than 10 per cent mentioned that their use of condoms derived from the advice they found in *Straight Talk*. Respondents who were sexually active and had not used condoms the last time they had sex most commonly gave the reason as 'not knowing about condoms', followed by 'not being able to access condoms'. Lack of knowledge of or access to condoms was four times more likely to be offered as reasons than 'trusting one's partner'. Commenting on these findings, Adamchack et al. (2007, 24), again suggest that following the introduction of ABC, *Straight Talk* had 'downplayed the discussion of condoms in the past few years, and these figures could be a reflection of that approach'.

Teachers are given some information about condom use in their teaching materials about HIV prevention, but interviews with teachers identified that they were encouraged not to mention condoms in their classroom teaching (Human Rights Watch, 2005). Given this, predictably, young people participating in Bell's research (conducted between 2002 and 2006) reported that the information they received about HIV in schools entailed either no messages about condoms or confusing messages: they frequently reported that, when the topic was raised, condoms were presented as appropriate for married people, alongside hormonal contraception, which they were taught could render them infertile if used prior to marriage.

In conducting his fieldwork in rural Uganda (personal communication), Stephen Bell noted that older people remembered their involvement in their communities' early HIV-prevention efforts in the form of community Resistance Councils (discussed above). They remembered community leaders visiting their houses and convening gatherings for collective discussion and education. It appears that, whereas early HIV-prevention efforts had engaged communities, current ones do not.

The provision of condoms in Uganda became an issue in the year after PEPFAR's introduction. In 2004 Uganda induced a condom shortage by recalling imported condoms on the basis of quality questions (prompted by complaints about the condoms' *smell* rather than breakage) and by instituting a policy of pre- and post-shipment testing of imported condoms, delaying their distribution (Human Rights Watch, 2005). Ongoing problems with condom distribution were clearly evident in 2010 and 2012 (Uganda AIDS Commission, 2010; 2012). The sheer numbers of condoms being distributed in Uganda declined steadily between 2007 and 2011 (see Figure 2.4 below).

Provider	NUMBER OF CONDOMS			
	2007/08	2008/09	2009/10	2010/11
Public				
MoH	80,999,148	51,596,150	61,292,338	35,000,000
Private				
MSI	18,227,232	15,786,120	18,834,438	8,786,301
PACE	2,616,150	6,047,250	4,012,710	8,051,700
UHMG	16,536,519	8,044,740	17,449,790	17,024,840
Total	118,379,049	81,474,260	101,589,276	68,862,841

Figure 2.4 Annual procurement and distribution of male condoms in Uganda (2007–2011).
Source: Uganda AIDS Commission (2012, 34).

More recently, the 2014 report states that, with respect to the preceding 12 months, '187 million male condoms have been procured and 101,729,000 sent out of warehouses' (Uganda AIDS Commission, 2014, 13). However, rather than aim for condoms to be available in outlets 100 per cent of the time, the report holds to a target to increase 'the availability of condoms in randomly selected outlets from 45% to 60%' (2014, 67).

Uganda's government reporting also evidences difficulties with envisaging who might use these condoms. Despite the fact that incidence is acknowledged to have risen, the National Priority Action Plan 2011/2012–2012/2013 (Uganda AIDS Commission, 2011, 5) aims to promote safe sex by '[e]xpand[ing] provision of HIV education for key populations [by] focusing on reduction of multiple sexual partnerships, cross-generational, transactional and early sex using curricular, life skills and peer network channels'. There is no gesture here towards the importance of addressing the fact that nearly half the seroconversions in adults are happening within marriage/cohabitating relationships (relationships still defined as 'non-risky sexual encounters' within the terminology of Ugandan reporting). This same plan does acknowledge the lack of effort to promote condoms for 'risky sexual encounters' (5), with a target of increasing the '[p]ercentage of randomly selected retail outlets and service delivery points that have condoms in stock increase from 45% to 60%' (4), (the unaltered target repeated three years later in the 2014 Country report) and a commitment to promote condoms using an unspecified 'mix of channels' and with a particular focus on 'urban areas and HIV hotspots' (5).

Perhaps not surprisingly, there are indications that condom use is declining – or declining amongst those whom are imagined to have cause to use them, being neither abstinent nor 'faithful' (see Figure 2.5). The 2012 Country report looks at condom use on the part of people 'with 2 or more partners' – excluding monogamous couples, married or not. We see a sharp decline in the use of condoms 'in last sexual encounter' from 51 per cent to 13.7 per cent between 2004/5 and 2011. Equally concerning is the defensive

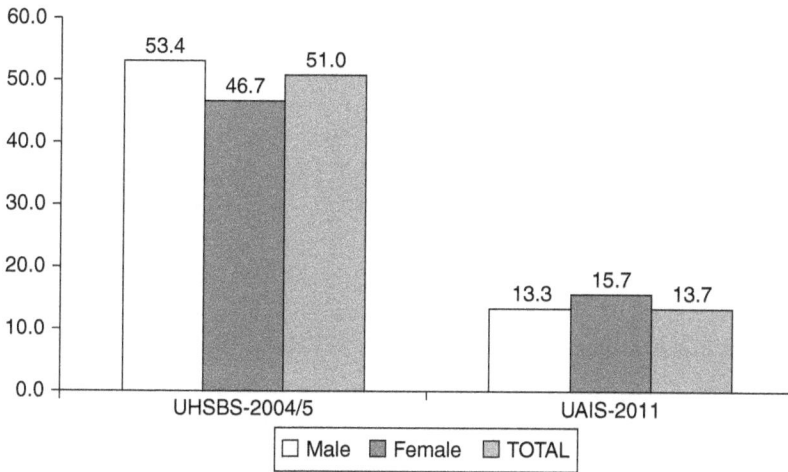

Figure 2.5 Percentage of people with 2+ partners using condoms during 'last sexual intercourse' by gender.
Source: Uganda AIDS Commission (2012, 33).

and misleading national reporting of this figure when it is broken down into age groups: 'The decline for those 15–29 was not very pronounced (52.7 to 30.2)' (2012, 33), when the decline is indeed large.

Trends of consistent condom use with regular or casual partners are impossible to come by. This is because[7] reporting of condom use is pre-framed by the ABC mentality of condoms as a last resort – to be used only by people who are not abstinent or faithful. So, although the 2010, 2012 and 2014 country reports foreground that transmission between regular partners is a significant part of rising incidence, people in such relationships are not being asked about safe sex using condoms, unless they report having multiple partners. Furthermore, survey respondents are not being asked to differenti-ate between condom use with different categories of partners, or about the consistency of their condom use. Furthermore, although detailed informa-tion about condom *access* was collected in the DHS in 2000–2001, 2006 and 2011 (Uganda Bureau of Statistics, 2001, 2007, 2012), since the 2003 intro-duction of PEPFAR funding to Uganda, it is *no longer being reported*. In each year, DHS respondents were asked (a) if they knew of sources where con-doms were available, and (b) if they could actually access condoms. However, being able to access a condom was only reported in 2000–2001 (in 2001 only 36.2 per cent of women 15–49 thought they could actually get a condom, and about 40 per cent of younger women, 15–24). The 2006 and 2011 DHS do not report the data collected.[8]

HIV testing

The picture regarding HIV testing is a very different from that of condom use. Indeed, the Ugandan uptake of HIV testing in the past decade is notable (Uganda Bureau of Statistics, 2001; 2007; 2012). In 2000–2001 only 12 per cent of adult men and 8 per cent of adult women aged 15–49 years had been tested for HIV. Five years later, 21 per cent of men and 25 per cent of women knew their status following a HIV test. And by 2011, 52 per cent of men and 71 per cent of women had tested and received results. Although promoting testing as a means of HIV prevention has been widely supported since the early 2000s, evidence for its effectiveness as a means of HIV prevention is lacking. A large-scale study undertaken in Zimbabwe by proponents of voluntary counselling and testing (VCT) found that knowledge of one's positive status was linked with safer sexual practices (Sherr et al., 2007); however, testing negative was associated with increases in some 'risky' sexual behaviours. The mechanism connecting these measures was not elucidated. It could be that knowledge of one's status is shared, and that two negative people make decisions based on this, or it could be that the relief of testing negative entails a sense of invulnerability, or affirms a sense of luck in having evaded the virus so far. In Chapter 5, we discuss the role that VCT has played in privatising discussions about HIV, relegating HIV prevention to being a matter for clinical one-on-one consultations, or clinician and couple conversations, rather than open, public discussion. But, here we want to note that in the late 1980s to early 1990s, when there was broad public discussion HIV, many people were aware of knowing HIV positive people (and most diagnoses would have been based on symptoms rather than a HIV test). As HIV testing became increasingly common among Ugandans, people were more inclined to see HIV status as a private matter. HIV prevention has become more vertically organised, and HIV incidence has risen.

Conclusions

Examining the two moments in the Ugandan epidemic reveals how HIV-prevention efforts embraced by the Ugandan government since the early 2000s have undermined the initial successes – that is, public discussion and debate that engaged people with the ideas that HIV was everyone's problem and that every citizen was responsible for HIV prevention, rather than being a moral issue that only demands the attention of those who fail to avoid 'risky' behaviour. While public health researchers debated 'evidence' of the success of Uganda's massive social experiment, the social terrain of the experiment radically changed: HIV became more private. Today, didactic, moralistic messages, the privatisation associated with moves to increase the role of the clinic in HIV prevention and the lack of information about what Ugandans are doing puts them at risk.

Delaying sex, reducing the number of sexual partners and using condoms were effective prevention methods because they came out of community discussion and engagement. Since then, abstinence and fidelity have been imposed by major funders and embraced by some in Ugandan public health for reasons that include their own evangelical agendas and the practical purposes of providing access to treatment (Meinert & Reynolds, 2014). Without public discussion and a sense of what Ugandans think matters to them, successful prevention in the form of Uganda's social vaccine is being eroded.

It is possible that the past 'successful strategies' may no longer be effective, because the social terrain of the HIV epidemic has changed. A recent study by Green et al. (2013) demonstrates that Ugandans now perceive HIV as a treatable chronic disease not unlike malaria. Biomedical developments in the form of effective treatment and better access to treatment, but also biomedical moves in prevention technologies, mean that HIV is now being seen differently. It is also likely that changes to the social and sexual practices of Ugandans – such as marriage at a later age – may be shaped by educational and economic opportunities and aspirations, and may trigger changes in the meanings of HIV. Knowing your epidemic involves understanding the social *as it changes*. Despite the fact that 'what worked in Uganda' has been discussed to the point of 'Uganda fatigue' (Green & Ruark, 2011; Green et al., 2013), these discussions have largely missed the fact that HIV-prevention policy worked because it harnessed and fuelled social mobilisation that was already happening. Furthermore, they missed this at a critical time in the global epidemic, when the moral agendas of cashed-up funders not only stopped engaging with some of the social changes that were occurring in Uganda, but fuelled efforts to actively counter them. The result was to close down the discussion and debate (the social vaccine) that marked and explained Uganda's early successes. The mismatch between current HIV prevention in Uganda and the fact that 43 per cent of adult HIV infections are estimated as occurring in monogamous relationships evidences the failure of HIV-prevention efforts to continue to engage with Ugandans' social practices.

Chapter 3

THE AUSTRALIAN PARTNERSHIP

We now turn to a very different country, Australia. Although a country with a quite dissimilar epidemic, it also initially responded successfully to the threat of HIV via what Low-Beer and Stoneburner refer to as a 'social vaccine'. However, as in Uganda, there has been a recent increase in HIV incidence, and in this chapter we seek an answer to the question, Why? This chapter traces 'three moments' in the Australian epidemic: the early years, 1983–1997; the years that followed the advent of successful treatments (ART) in 1996 (1998–2009); and the turn to treatment for prevention after 2009.

The epidemic was and continues to be very different from what we have described as occurring in Uganda: Australia's is a 'concentrated' epidemic that affects gay and homosexually active men. Although sex workers, people who inject drugs and the general population are also at risk of HIV, transmission has been minimal in these populations as compared with the gay and homosexually active population, as shown in Figure 3.1 below.

The spread of HIV among people who inject drugs was curtailed by quick action (Madden & Wodak, 2014), and transmission among the heterosexual population was minimised by the responses of sex workers (Bates & Berg, 2014), school authorities (Jones & Mitchell, 2014), Indigenous Australians (Ward et al., 2014) and the Australian national and state governments (Persson et al., 2014). The relatively sustained success of these Australian HIV-prevention efforts can be attributed to a wide range of actions by communities and networks supported by government. A detailed account of these responses is given by Mindel & Kippax (2013) and in a special issue of *AIDS Education & Prevention* edited by Aggleton & Kippax (2014).

As shown in Figure 3.1, HIV incidence in Australia peaked among gay and other homosexually active men (men who have sex with men, MSM) in 1987–1988, then declined rapidly until 1997–1998 and then increased with some fluctuations, including a large increase post-2011. In other populations, HIV incidence peaked in about 1994–1995 and then also rapidly declined until 1998. Since that time there have been small fluctuations, but there has been no substantial increase of HIV transmission among Indigenous Australians, people who inject drugs or sex workers and their clients. However there has been a small but significant increase among heterosexuals in minority ethnic communities and among a mobile population in Western Australia working on a fly-in and fly-out basis in a range of industries (Persson et al., 2014).

As the HIV epidemic in Australia was, and continues to be, largely driven by male-to-male sexual transmission, the remainder of this chapter focuses, although not exclusively, on three moments that capture gay men's HIV-prevention response: the dramatic decline in HIV incidence in the early years (Holt, 2014; Race 2014a), the first increase in HIV incidence in 1997–1998, and the second increase of around 10 per cent, evident since 2011 (see Figure 3.1).

The First Moment: The Early Years (1983–1997)

In Australia the first case of AIDS was diagnosed in 1982 in a gay man in Sydney, and between 1982 and 1985 HIV spread rapidly, with an estimated 4,500 people infected, predominantly in the gay community in Sydney and to a lesser extent in Melbourne. Gay and other homosexually active men remain the largest group affected by HIV in Australia. HIV transmission continues

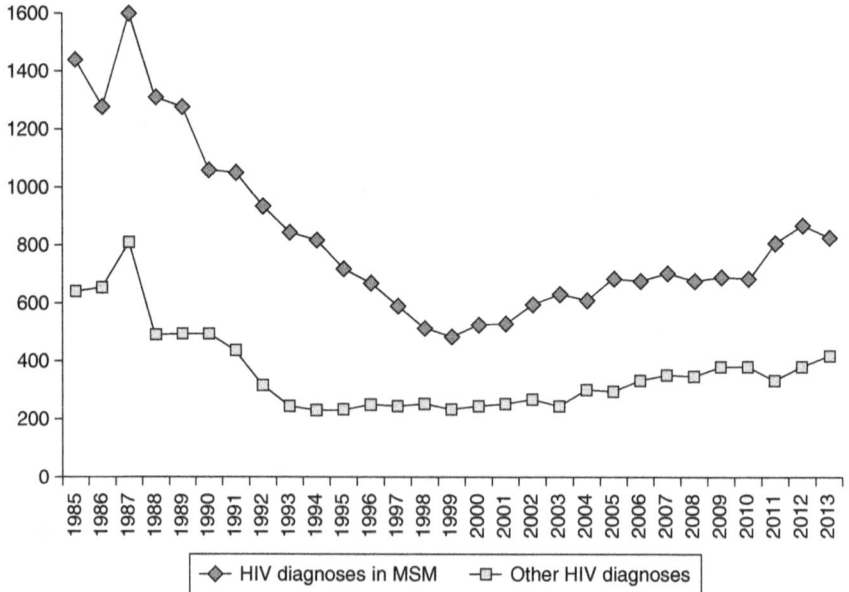

Figure 3.1 HIV diagnoses in Australia per year (1985–2013).

Source: Data derived from the HIV, Viral Hepatitis, STIs in Australia, Annual Surveillance Report, 2014, the Kirby Institute.

to occur mainly through sexual contact between men and, in the period 2009–2013, accounted for 64 per cent of newly diagnosed HIV infections (or 67% if MSM who also inject drugs are included) and 85 per cent (or 88% inclusive of MSM who inject drugs) of newly acquired infections (Kirby Institute, 2014, 11).

The majority of the early infections took place at a time when relatively little was known about HIV. In consequence, men within the gay community and their friends were forced to look to their own resources – organising politically and socially and drawing upon experience both at home and elsewhere in the world, especially that of their gay peers in San Francisco and New York – to mount their HIV response. Given that homosexual behaviour between men remained illegal in many states in Australia until the mid-1980s and into the 1990s in Queensland and Tasmania, these early gay community struggles were not easy. The challenges of responding to HIV arose at around the same time the gay community in Australia was organising and becoming politically active around discrimination against homosexually active men.

Gay community responses to HIV were supported by the Australian federal and state governments. Australia was fortunate at that moment to have a health minister who was a political scientist, Neal Blewett. What Blewett understood was that HIV, in particular HIV prevention, requires that the key players (community activists, clinicians and other public health workers, researchers, educators, policymakers) understand and harness people's ways of actively striving to deal with HIV in their everyday lives. It involves encouraging and enabling people to transform their sexual lives. He rejected the 'contain and control' model of traditional public health with its emphasis on identification of the infected, contact tracing and, if necessary quarantine. Instead, acting on his understanding that HIV prevention is essentially about social transformation at the meso- and macro-social levels, he had government invest in peer-led education and community-building programmes and orchestrated a cost-sharing arrangement with the states, stipulating that at least half of the AIDS funding was to be spent on prevention.

Not only did the federal and state governments support the initiatives of communities, but they built strong links with communities at risk of HIV. Also early in the epidemic, the Australian government secured the blood supply, established three national centres in HIV biomedical, clinical and epidemiological and social research and mounted a number of television and other media information campaigns to inform all Australians about HIV. AIDS (as it was then known) was from the start understood as requiring a broad-based, multi-faceted and collaborative response with the national strategic approach to HIV and AIDS being based on a partnership between governments,

communities, clinicians and biomedical, epidemiological and social researchers (Bowtell, 2008; Mindel & Kippax, 2013).

The early response of gay community

As in the early days in Uganda, the early success was a function of a 'social
vaccine'. The HIV response took root in the everyday social relations of gay
communities and networks via a community communication process. This
communication process was not only a response to the ever-present illness,
AIDS, it was also a call to prevent HIV transmission. There was talk about,
and the development of, support networks for those living and dying with
AIDS, and talk about how to maintain one's HIV-negative status and prevent
the spread of HIV. HIV was palpably present, as was the case in Uganda, in
the period between 1985 and 1997 almost all HIV-negative or untested gay
men said they knew someone living with HIV (Kippax, Connell, Dowsett &
Crawford, 1993, 163), around 95 per cent in 1986 and around 90 per cent
in the years between 1993 and 1997. In 1986–1997 the proportion of HIV-
negative or untested gay men interviewed in Sydney who knew someone who
had died of AIDS was 61 per cent and the proportion of men caring for
someone with AIDS was 30 per cent. As men became ill, HIV became more
and more obvious, and illness and death were commonplace among friends
and colleagues. Funerals were daily events.

During this same period, gay communities were active in urging their members across Australia to use condoms. As well as taking up condoms, gay men
found safe ways to have unprotected sex, as documented by Holt (2014) in his
discussion of 'epistemic communities'. These safe-sex strategies were rapidly
built on and incorporated into HIV-prevention education and prevention programmes. As highlighted by Race (2014a), these strategies and the manner in
which they were evaluated provide a stark contrast to a more traditional public
health approach. It is of note that the majority of gay and other homosexually active men in Australia in this early period did not embrace abstinence or
monogamy – and indeed did not reduce the number of their sexual partners
(Kippax & Race, 2003). As well as adopting condoms – which, during this
period, approximately 70 per cent of men consistently used with their casual
sexual partners – they also developed a range of other strategies that they
believed reduced their risk of HIV transmission. These included negotiated
safety, withdrawal, positive–positive sex and strategic positioning.

What is important here is that these responses – and many of them reduced,
if not eradicated, risk of HIV transmission – came *from* the community. Compared with gay men with little or a loose attachment to the gay community, gay
men who were strongly engaged in gay-community activities were the first to

reduce the risk of HIV transmission (Kippax, Connell, Dowsett & Crawford, 1993). The early social researchers in Australia developed three measures of gay community engagement. The gay community involvement scale measured men's immersion in modern gay culture and politics: someone with a high score on this scale was likely to read a gay newspaper, patronise gay shops and businesses, go to a gay-identified doctor, attend gay functions (sporting, politi- cal, cultural) and be a member of one or more gay organisations. The social engagement scale measured social engagement with other gay men: men with high scores on this scale were likely to have many gay friends, spend much of their free time with gay men, and be someone for whom much of their social contact took place in gay bars and other gay venues. The third scale captured sexual engagement in the gay community: men with a high score on this scale had many casual sexual partners whom they sought at a wide range of sex venues, and frequently engaged in casual sex. The men who were attached to the gay community – sexually and socially – were those who were most likely to have adopted safe sexual practices, including condom use: the greater the attachment, the greater the likelihood that they had reduced their risk of HIV transmission via changes in their sexual practice. It is of interest to note here that men with minimal sexual engagement in the gay community had poor knowledge of safe sexual practices and were more likely to change the nature of their sexual relationships and move toward monogamy and celibacy.

The adoption of safe sexual strategies emerged out of the talk between gay men. While condom use was the most common form of risk reduction, other strategies emerged on the basis of what men understood from their reading of the biomedical literature, These strategies were identified and described by researchers and, if thought to be likely to reduce risk, were developed by educators in the AIDS councils and, with the support of government funding, were incorporated into gay community prevention campaigns. These strategies included 'negotiated safety' – a special form of what is now called 'serosorting'. 'Negotiated safety', which was first identified by researchers (Kippax et al., 1993, 1997), is a deliberate strategy on the part of men in committed/primary relationships. Such men, on the basis of knowing that their own and their regular sexual partner's HIV status was HIV-negative (through being tested), agreed to dispense with condoms within their relationships without necessarily giving up sex or anal intercourse outside relationships: the men agreeing to use condoms for anal intercourse outside of the primary relationship.

Negotiated safety was not a strategy imposed from the outside, but one that was grounded on an already-existing practice – that is, the practice of persons in regular committed relationships dispensing with condoms dur- ing sex in that relationship after informing each other of their negative HIV status. The safe adoption of such a strategy involves communication, talk,

familiarity and ease with one's sexual partner, as well as trust, but not necessarily fidelity. While withdrawal (another strategy that emerged from gay community) was not promoted, negotiated safety was promoted as a risk-reduction
strategy with the support of funding from the New South Wales government.
A health-promotion campaign was developed by educators within the AIDS
Council of New South Wales (ACON) and was run first in New South Wales
and then other states (Kinder, 1996; Kippax & Kinder, 2002). It has been
shown to be an effective HIV-prevention strategy among gay men in Australia
(Jin et al., 2008). The development of this community strategy and its proven
effectiveness in Australia demonstrate the importance of community engagement and involvement in HIV-prevention activities. Scientific knowledge,
both biomedical and social, was and continues to be taken up and socially
transformed by those most affected by the epidemic. Members of affected
communities acted collectively as agents taking up the challenge of HIV and
engaged with various pieces of knowledge and understandings – from the
medical and social sciences as well as from their own everyday experience – in
order to protect themselves, their partners and communities.

During this period, the Australian AIDS councils continued to produce
HIV-prevention education materials, based in the main on strategies developed by gay men (some of it sexually explicit) for distribution in gay media,
bars and sex venues. Some of it attracted adverse media attention but in the
main, the governments (state and federal) have continued to fund these education materials. These campaigns targeting gay men have been highly successful in raising awareness of HIV, stimulating debate and discussion within
gay community and increasing safe sexual practice. In a variety of ways, the
gay community – in its social, sexual and cultural forms – provided gay men
with a supportive environment that enabled them to produce risk-reduction
strategies and to negotiate safe sex. HIV transmission was radically reduced
(see Figure 3.2).

The Second Moment: What Happened to the
Social Vaccine (1998–2009)?

In 1997–1998 effective treatments became available, and those who had been
facing almost certain death no longer did. AIDS incidence amongst MSM
peaked in 1994–1995 and then dropped radically for the first time since the
start of the epidemic (see Figure 3.2).

Not only were dramatically fewer people dying of AIDS with an associated
remarkable absence of funerals for young men who had died of AIDS but,
also from 1997 onwards, HIV became less and less visible (see Table 3.1). Following the success of ART in preventing AIDS, the percentage of gay men in

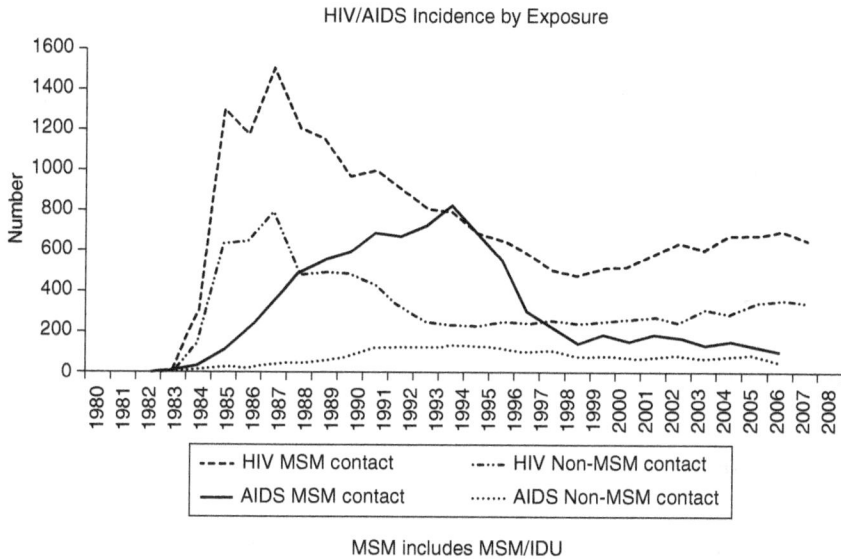

HIV/AIDS Incidence by Exposure

---- HIV MSM contact   ·--· HIV Non-MSM contact
—— AIDS MSM contact   ······ AIDS Non-MSM contact

MSM includes MSM/IDU

Figure 3.2 HIV/AIDS incidence by exposure (1982–2008).

Source: Data derived from the HIV, Viral Hepatitis, STIs in Australia, Annual Surveillance Report, 2009, the Kirby Institute.

Table 3.1 Forms of contact with HIV among non–HIV-positive men.

STUDY (date)	% Knowing PLHIV	% Knowing Someone Died of AIDS	% Knowing Someone Died last 12 months	% Caring for PLHIV/ AIDS
SAPA 86/7	99	61		30
SSS 91	99	90		55
SMASH 93	87		62	
SMASH 97	93		66	23
SMASH 98	90		55	20
HIM 2001	85	68	27	
HIM 2006	87		10	

Note: All data shown in this table derive from studies carried out in New South Wales. The data shown here are based on all non-positive (men who do not know their HIV status or who are HIV-negative) gay men living in Sydney who were interviewed at the time of the studies. The behavioural epidemiological studies included are: SAPA – Social Aspects of the Prevention of AIDS; SSS –Sustaining Safe Sex; SMASH – Sydney Men and Sexual Health; HIM – Health in Men.

Source: Data derived from research undertaken by the National Centre in HIV Social Research/ The Centre for Social Research in Health, the University of New South Wales, Australia.

Sydney who reported knowing someone who had died of AIDS in the previous 12 months dropped radically from 66 per cent in 1997 to 10 per cent in
2006. The proportion of people caring for those living with HIV/AIDS also
declined between 1986 and 1998: because of ART, very few people living
with HIV are now in need of care, and very few people are currently caring
for people with HIV/AIDS. With the advent of ART, HIV became a chronic
illness, an illness held in check and an illness with few visible symptoms. This
shift in visibility occurred despite the fact that the prevalence of HIV in Australia was higher in gay communities in the years following the introduction of
ART (1996) and continues to rise.

Decline in condom use

At the same time as HIV was becoming less visible among gay communities,
and certainly from 1998 onwards, there was a small but gradual increase in
HIV infections and, as HIV incidence increased, unprotected sex with sexual
partners increased: the proportion of men engaging in any unprotected anal
intercourse with casual sexual partners during this period increased by around
15 per cent, and with regular partners by around 10 per cent (see Figures 3.3
and 3.4).

As the large majority of men engaging in unprotected anal intercourse
with their regular partners were likely to have adopted the 'negotiated safety'
strategy, the increase in Figure 3.4 is not as troubling as the increase in unprotected anal intercourse with casual partners, since 'negotiated safety' has been

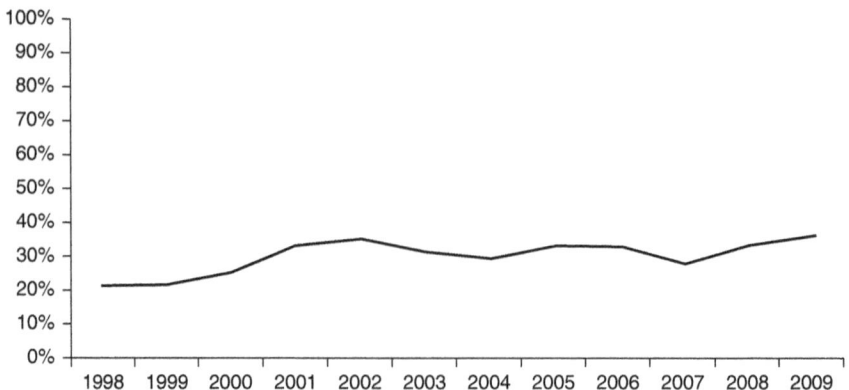

Figure 3.3 Proportion of men engaging in any unprotected anal intercourse with
casual partner(s) (1998–2009).

Source: Data derived from Gay Community Periodic Surveys (1998–2009), National Centre in
HIV Social Research, the University of New South Wales, Australia.

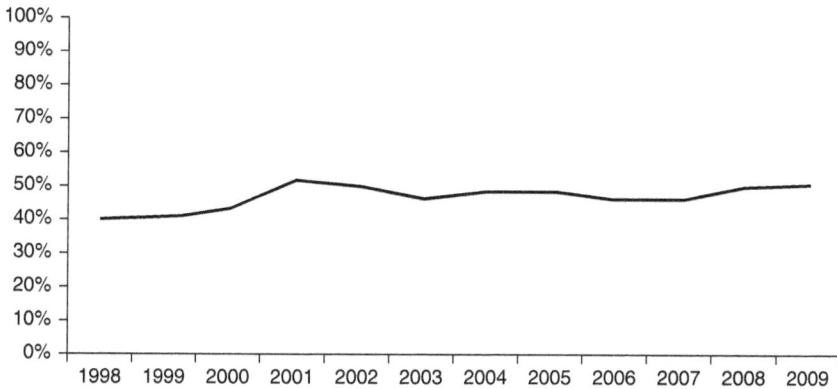

Figure 3.4 Proportion of men engaging in any unprotected anal intercourse with regular partner(s) (1998–2009).

Source: Data derived from Gay Community Periodic Surveys (1998–2009), National Centre in HIV Social Research, the University of New South Wales, Australia.

shown to be a relatively safe risk-reduction strategy. However, these two sets of data together indicate a general move away from condom use. The decline in condom use is most likely a function of a number of factors. One factor was the optimism – on the part of funding agencies as well as MSM – associated with HIV being understood as a chronic disease rather than a death sentence. Another related factor was the adoption by gay men of a number of risk-reduction strategies in which condoms play no part.

Optimism

The fact that there is now an effective treatment for HIV was cause for optimism. Not only did HIV become less visible on the streets of Australian cities with large gay communities, but there was a sense that between 1987 and the late 1990s the HIV-prevention response had been a success. However, since the end of the 1990s there has been a slow but significant increase in unprotected anal intercourse among gay and other homosexually active men as shown above in Figures 3.3 and 3.4. The significant increase in sexual risk behaviour among gay men in Australia parallels that documented in the United States (Denning et al., 2000; Ekstrand et al., 2000), the Netherlands (Dukers et al., 2000), and England (Dodds et al., 2000). It is likely that the decline in knowing someone with HIV/AIDS influenced the observed increase in unprotected anal intercourse, and the uptake of the condom-free, harm-reduction strategies was shaped by optimism. Fear of HIV infection diminished in gay communities across Australia and, as we discuss below, HIV prevention began to drop off the community agenda. As HIV became less visible and deaths were reduced to near zero, there was less talk and discussion of HIV: HIV as a chronic illness is easier to contemplate than as a cause of death.

Although in Australia in the early to mid-1990s there was no evidence of a simple causal relationship between knowing someone with HIV and adopting safe sex,[1] over time and certainly by the late 1990s findings from studies began to indicate a significant relationship between gay men's sexual risk-taking operationalised as unprotected anal intercourse with casual partners (UAIC) and optimism in the context of new HIV treatments (Van de Ven et al., 1999). In this and following studies, risk-taking was independently related to optimism: men who were more optimistic about HIV treatment advances were more likely to engage in UAIC (Van de Ven et al., 2000, 2002). Although in these studies, mean scores on the HIV optimism scale tended toward scepticism, men with higher optimism scores, both those living with HIV and those who were HIV-negative, were more likely to report UAIC. It seems likely that as AIDS and death receded from the collective consciousness of the gay community and optimism grew, the condom culture, which developed in the mid-1980s, was undermined. Although there was an ongoing attempt on the part of gay men to reduce risk, some of the strategies adopted, which we discuss below, are not as safe as condom use.

On the basis of an effective treatment in the form of ART, gay men were urged to test and to test frequently. And although before the advent of effective treatments some AIDS councils were reluctant to endorse testing, their views changed when treatments became effective: the councils then urged their constituents to test. So, although 30 per cent of men in an early study in 1986–1987 had not tested for HIV, by 1991 only 13 per cent remained untested (Kippax, Connell, Dowsett & Crawford, 1993). This proportion of untested men fell to 10 per cent in 1998 and remained at approximately that level up until 2009 (see Figure 3.5).

Men also began to test more frequently (see Figure 3.6), although the increase – from just below 60 per cent in 1998 to just under 70 per cent in 2009 – was not as high as many in public health would have liked.

Knowledge of one's own test results and the expectation that sexual partners might also know their HIV status enabled the emergence of new risk-reduction strategies. In Australia, as mentioned, negotiated safety was produced by HIV-negative men in the gay community, promoted with funding from government and adopted by many as a way of engaging safely in unprotected anal intercourse with their seroconcordant negative regular partners.

Over time, although not promoted, it was evident that gay men, both HIV-positive and HIV-negative, often sought out partners of the same serostatus and in doing so often abandoned condoms. In the United States and

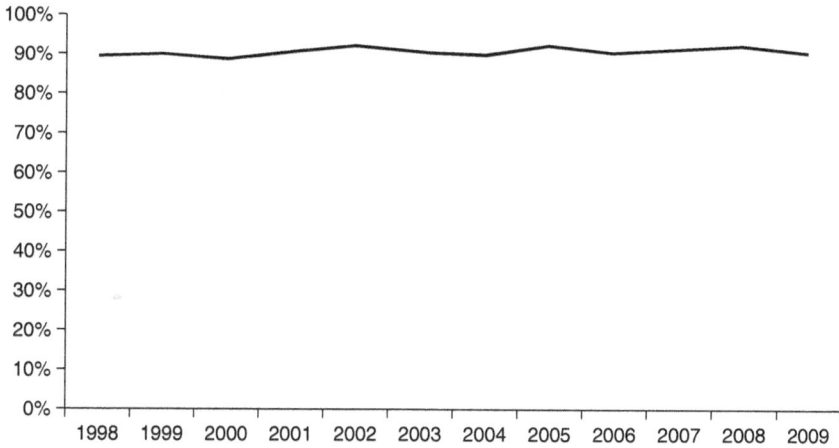

Figure 3.5 Proportion of non-positive gay men in Australia ever tested (1998–2009).

Source: Data derived from Gay Community Periodic Surveys (1998–2009), National Centre in HIV Social Research, the University of New South Wales, Australia.

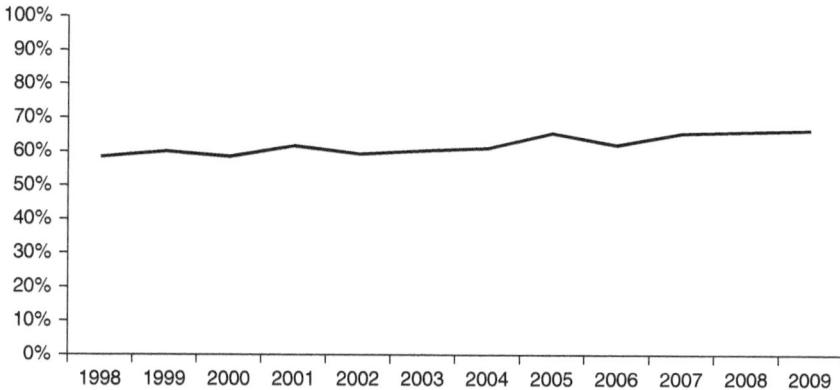

Figure 3.6 Proportion of non-positive gay men in Australia tested in the previous 12 months (1998–2009).

Source: Data derived from Gay Community Periodic Surveys (1998–2009), National Centre in HIV Social Research, the University of New South Wales, Australia.

elsewhere, this practice – a practice of abandoning condoms with known or assumed seroconcordant sexual partners – was referred to as 'serosorting'. Although the term 'serosorting' was initially used to describe the patterning of sexual encounters on the basis of the HIV-test status of their sexual partners, the use of the term to describe a deliberate HIV-prevention strategy on the part of gay men seeking partners of the same serostatus took hold in the early 2000s. Suarez & Miller (2001) published a review of strategies used by gay men to reduce HIV transmission, particularly when engaging in unprotected anal intercourse (UAI). Serosorting was defined as discussing HIV status with potential partners (particularly casual partners) and limiting UAI to seroconcordant partners. It was grouped with negotiated safety as 'rational risk-taking'. Suarez & Miller acknowledged that serosorting was an attempt to reduce harm when having UAI, but highlighted the strategy's heavy reliance on accurate knowledge of HIV status, effective HIV disclosure and honesty. Studies in Australia (Jin et al., 2009) demonstrated that while negotiated safety (with regular partners) was not associated with increased risk of HIV transmission, serosorting with casual partners carried some risk.

As well as negotiated safety and its more general form, serosorting, other strategies to minimise risk of HIV-transmission based on medical knowledge and advances also emerged from within the gay community. One such strategy was 'strategic positioning' where, in known or potentially serodiscordant relationships, HIV-negative men take up the insertive position and HIV-positive men the receptive position in anal intercourse without the use of condoms (Rosengarten, Race & Kippax, 2000; Van de Ven et al., 2004). Another was 'reliance on the undetectable viral load' of one's HIV-positive sexual partner (Van de Ven et al., 2005). In this strategy in a serodiscordant relationship in which it is known or assumed that the HIV-positive partner has an undetectable viral load, unprotected anal intercourse is considered safe or 'safe enough'. This strategy was adopted by a small number of gay men in Australia ahead of findings demonstrating that 'treatment as prevention' (which is now commonly referred to as TasP) may be effective under certain conditions: the Swiss Consensus Statement (Vernazza et al., 2008), the modelling work by Granich et al. (2009) and the HPTN randomised controlled trial (RCT) of TasP (Cohen et al., 2011).

These strategies have become part of the armoury of HIV prevention for gay men in Australia. Some of these are more effective in reducing harm than others, and they give gay men a number of choices. However, choices also produce indecision and uncertainty, as Prestage et al. (2013) discuss in their paper titled, 'It's hard to know what is a risky or not a risky decision'. Notwithstanding such dilemmas, gay men use, and will continue to use, medical and other knowledge to fashion prevention strategies that, although they are not 100 per cent risk-free, can be built into their everyday lives and can be sustained. All the above strategies were typically associated with the abandoning of condoms and, although their adoption reduces the risk of HIV transmission to *some* degree, HIV infections increased during the period post-1997. Consistent condom use appears to be a more effective strategy than using non–condom-based risk-reduction strategies.

The increasing medicalisation of HIV prevention

Increasingly during this time period, factors other than optimism were also in play. As treatment became increasingly (and understandably) important, and with the accompanying greater HIV response emphasis on HIV testing, the clinic took up a more and more central position – not only with regard to treatment but also to prevention. HIV testing was urged by bodies such as the World Health Organization (WHO) and the Joint United Nations Programme on HIV/AIDS (UNAIDS) in the early 2000s and was promoted as a prevention measure as well as a way into care and treatment if one tested HIV-positive (Kippax, 2006).

A number of claims were made, and of importance here was the claim that the clinic is a site of effective prevention education. Voluntary counselling and testing (VCT) were positioned by many as the gateway to prevention. It was argued that knowing one's test status would strengthen safe sex: HIV-negative people would act to ensure that they remained so, while HIV-positive people, knowing that they were positive, would not engage in unsafe sexual behaviour. The accumulating evidence does not support this: while most HIV-positive people do act to protect their sexual partners (Marks et al., 2006), HIV-negative people do not reduce their risk behaviour. The authors of a meta-analysis of studies conducted between 1985 and 1997 concluded that counselling and testing are not an effective primary prevention strategy for uninfected people (Weinhardt et al., 1999) and more recent evidence from Zimbabwe (Sherr et al. 2007) indicates that not only is counselling and testing ineffective for people who test HIV-negative, but that counselling and testing may have the serious unintended consequence of increasing risk behaviours.

Not only was testing not effective as prevention, but the move to position the clinic as a site of prevention had a number of outcomes. As we describe in Chapters 4 and 5, the clinic has an individualising tendency: illness is privatised and community input into prevention is jeopardised, albeit unintentionally. However, here we focus mainly on the more-immediate outcomes. The emphasis on testing reinforced moves among gay men to serosort as they sought sexual partners, and governments and non-governmental organisations slowly began to focus resources on testing and treatment rather than on prevention.

Positive prevention

At the same time that researchers, the Australian gay community and public health organisations were coming to recognise and appraise developments in the HIV risk-reduction strategies being devised by MSM, the wider (overseas and international) discussion of HIV prevention was being shaped by a new emphasis on 'positive prevention'. This policy was first introduced in 2003 when the Centers for Disease Control (CDC) in the United States announced a national initiative focused on preventing new infections by working with persons diagnosed with HIV and their partners (CDC, 2003). Since that time, internationally focused guidance on 'positive prevention' has been developed by UNAIDS, the International HIV/AIDS Alliance and WHO (see for example GNP+, UNAIDS (2011). Although these organisations' more recent policy documents have emphasised that preventing HIV transmission is a shared responsibility of all, irrespective of HIV status, and 'positive prevention' was not explicitly embraced in Australia, the international attention produced some confusion. In this climate, for some men the production of a condom prior to sex was understood as 'I am HIV-positive' while, for others, its absence was read as 'I am HIV-negative' (Rosengarten, Race & Kippax, 2000). In this sense, the meaning of condom use was shifting in this period. Research on the early uptake of condoms by gay and other homosexually active men foregrounded the role of condoms in shaping social relations between them that entailed 'new forms of mutual responsibility and autonomy' (Weeks, 1998, 44). The meaning ascribed to condoms with their early adoption in the 1980s and early 1990s was that condom use signalled an expression of care (for oneself and others) and one's affiliation with the gay community. Condom use was inclusive of positive and negative men. Discussion of 'positive prevention', however, shatters this inclusiveness.

Shifts in funding

In the period 1997–2009 there was also a shift from the innovative crisis-driven time of the early epidemic to a more traditional and institutionalised response (Brown et al., 2014). The focus on treatment and testing had an impact on government funding, and there was a shift in funding away from prevention and toward treatment. Notwithstanding the evidence that counselling and testing is not an effective primary prevention strategy (rather testing is best positioned as an adjunct to prevention), within the context of the increased focus on treatments, spending on HIV-prevention waned.

This shift in funding took place at the same time as the partnership between community organisations such as the AIDS councils and the state governments began to change, although not in all states. An analysis of three Australian states' responses to increases in new HIV diagnoses in gay men indicated that there were differences in the ways the partnership functioned, the types of prevention strategies supported, the proportional size of the prevention workforce and the financial investment in prevention (Fairley et al., 2008; Bernard et al., 2008; NSW Department of Health, 2007). The comparison between the states indicated that in New South Wales the higher per-capita investment was a contributing factor in stabilising HIV incidence in that state – at least until 2012 (see below), as compared with the continuing significant increases in incidence in both Victoria and Queensland (Bernard et al., 2008). Compared with the partnership in New South Wales, the partnership in Victoria was viewed as poor, with requests in the early 2000s for more funding to be spent on prevention ignored. In Queensland, too, it was noted that the response to increases in HIV was slow. Furthermore, although Queensland funding was reasonably stable, media campaigns were perceived to be highly censored and conservative.

Any interpretation of, and response to, the epidemiological trends in HIV notifications and increases in unsafe sexual practice needs to take into account the nature of the partnership between government/public health and community and the resource differences. Partnership and resourcing are central to ensuring that supporting and working with gay communities to address HIV prevention is done in the most effective manner. The responses of communities to HIV risk and the highly sophisticated strategies deployed by gay men to reduce risk need to be understood and acknowledged by governments if a safe-sex culture is to be sustained.

Changing community

The gay community was also evolving and changing, and continues to do so. While, in the early 1980s, AIDS changed the face of gay communities, in the following 20 to 30 years gay communities changed again – in part in response to the changing face of HIV/AIDS. In many ways, as described by Altman (2013, 111), HIV contributed to the mainstreaming of gay life and overtime – as HIV became a largely chronic manageable condition, the centrality of AIDS as an organising trope for the gay community declined. HIV is no longer a central issue for young gay men coming out and entering the gay community. Similarly, Holt (2011) identified the ways that the galvanising effect of HIV on some gay men's sense of community is located in the past.

At the same time, the pathways that MSM identify and cultivate with regard to 'coming out' today are different, especially with respect to the orientation they take toward the gay community (Rowe & Dowsett, 2008). Altman comments: 'The last two decades have seen a steady growth of social acceptance and the breaking down of taboos, but whether this means that sexuality has become irrelevant to identity and politics remains an open question' (Altman, 2013, 150). Reynolds (2007) agrees: 'I believe that the phase of gay life which was centred upon inner-city communities and a discrete, highly commercial gay identity – the age of the uber-gay – has had its cultural moment. [...] Gay life [...] is an auxiliary of self. [...] We are more than who we choose to bed' (193–194).

Nonetheless, sexual practice remains central to many, and there are now many more ways to 'hook-up'. One of the significant changes in this regard concerns the ways in which sexual partners are sought. Digital devices – in particular the hook-up devices of smart phone applications – are affording novel ways of arranging sex, intimacy and sexual community with their own qualities and limitations (Race, 2014b, 2015). Race argues that the sexual relations made possible by these devices – the typical forms of connection and estrangement – are key, not only for understanding, but for generating new forms of sexual community among gay men (2015, 269); modes of connection whereby declarations of HIV status can precede online contact and discussions of status can occur online, prompting thought about the emergence of new ways of responding to HIV risk-reduction.

The Third Moment: Treatment as Prophylaxis and Prevention (2010–2014)

It may be premature to define a third moment, but a 10 per cent increase in HIV incidence among gay and other homosexually active men in Australia during the period 2010–2013 warrants scrutiny. In the period 2010–2014, treatment in the form of pre-exposure prophylaxis (PrEP) was being trialled for prevention of HIV transmission among gay men, as was TasP. At the same time as fewer and fewer men reported knowing anyone with HIV – 31 per cent of gay men interviewed in 2013 said that they knew no one living with HIV (Martin Holt, personal communication) compared with almost no men in 1987 and around 15 per cent in the mid-2000s (see Table 3.1 above) – there was more and more optimistic talk of ART as prevention. The medicalisation of prevention has gained momentum.

PrEP

Pre-exposure prophylaxis comes in two forms: topical microbicides and oral drugs. Vaginal microbicides have been developed and trialled but have shown disappointingly relatively low efficacy of 39 per cent (Abdool Karim et al., 2010). Gay men have indicated interest in using rectal microbicides, and rectal microbicide candidates are currently undergoing clinical trial assessment. In a recent study in Australia (Murphy et al., 2015) fewer than 20 per cent of gay men expressed strong interest in rectal microbicides, and interest in using microbicides was independently associated with having a greater self-perceived likelihood of becoming HIV-positive, having any unprotected anal sex with casual partners in the previous six months, and ever having received post-exposure prophylaxis.

PrEP in the form of oral drugs has been trialled in both heterosexual and homosexual populations – with mixed results in heterosexual populations, particularly in women (Van der Straten et al., 2012). When trialled in gay male populations, however, efficacy has been consistently relatively high, between 42 per cent and 99 per cent, depending on adherence (Grant et al., 2010). Notwithstanding the mixed results, in May 2014 the CDC and the US Public Health Service released new clinical guidelines recommending that health-care providers consider PrEP for 'patients at substantial risk for HIV infection' (CDC, 2014). Within the US guidelines, those considered at substantial risk include a 'gay or bisexual man who has had sex without a condom or been diagnosed with a sexually transmitted infection within the past six months'.

Although PrEP is not currently available in Australia, studies among gay and other homosexually active men (Holt et al., 2012, 2014a) indicate that gay men are cautiously optimistic about using PrEP and that a minority are willing to use PrEP. Those willing to do so are more likely to engage in unprotected anal intercourse with their casual sexual partners than those who are not willing.

Treatment as prevention

Around the same time, TasP became a hot topic. Based on observational data, a group of Swiss biomedical scientists released what is known as the Swiss Consensus Statement (2008), which declared that treatment of HIV greatly reduces the risk of HIV transmission between cohabiting heterosexual serodis-cordant partners, where the HIV-positive partner is on ART: ART reduces the HIV-positive person's viral load to an undetectable or very low level and thus reduces the likelihood of onward transmission to his or her partner to near zero. Initially, there was notably little discussion of the Swiss statement. However policy and programme interest began to develop following the publication of a mathematical modelling study (Granich et al., 2009) that suggested suppression of viral load on a population scale could have dramatic effects on HIV transmission. Two years later, the results of an RCT – the HPTN052 study by Cohen et al. (2011) – confirmed the finding for stable cohabiting heterosexual couples in serodiscordant relationships and calculated that treatment reduced the risk of transmission by 96 per cent.[2] Findings from a study focused on sero-discordant male couples shows that treatment of the HIV-positive partner also prevents HIV transmission, with a maximum of 1 per cent per year chance of transmission from any anal sex (Rodger et al., 2014). Taken together these findings were hailed by many as heralding 'the end of the epidemic' and promising claims were made about the *population impact* of TasP. The labelling of the New South Wales[3] HIV Strategy Document 2012–2015 as 'A New Era' echoes such claims about the promises of TasP: HIV TasP is positioned as the 'new era' (Gale et al., 2014). While maintaining safe sex is a priority, its major focus is in treating, testing and the uptake of treatment among those who are found to be HIV-positive (NSW Ministry of Health, 2012).

In the absence of evidence to establish the real world effectiveness of TasP, it is important to note that according to some modellers – for example, Wilson (2012) – that if Granich et al. (2009) were correct, the world should *already* be witnessing downturns in HIV infections, especially in places such as Australia, where testing rates are high and access to ART is guaranteed for citizens and permanent residents. Furthermore, the early observational data on which the Swiss Consensus Statement was based, and the findings from the RCTs (Cohen et al., 2011; Rodger et al., 2014) were based on serodiscordant *cohabiting couples*, both heterosexual and homosexual: so, although, in the absence of risk compensation it is likely that the population impact will not be negligible, the real-world impact remains unknown.

The impact that TasP and its rhetoric – described by some as 'medical triumphalism' – are likely to have on broader prevention efforts on HIV transmission has yet to unfold and be assessed. And, although gay men in Australia express some scepticism about TasP (Holt et al., 2014b), it does appear that condom use has further declined. For instance, behavioural surveys (see Figure 3.7) of Australian gay and other homosexually active men conducted since 1998

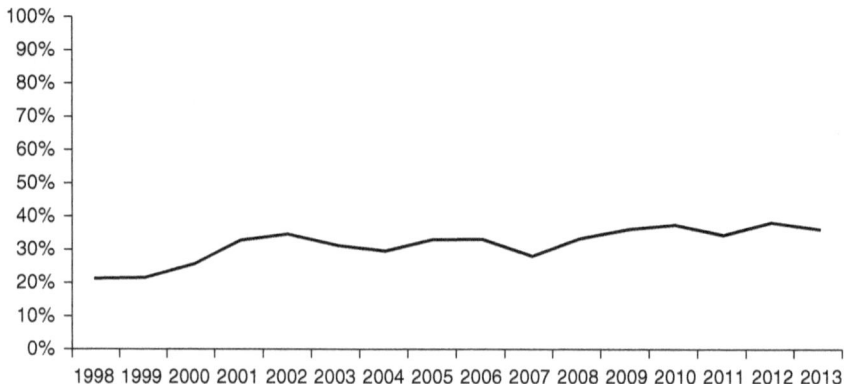

Figure 3.7 Proportion of men engaging in any unprotected anal intercourse with casual partner(s) (1998–2013).

Source: Data derived from Gay Community Periodic Surveys (1998–2013), National Centre in HIV Social Research/Centre for Social Research in Health, the University of New South Wales, Australia.

indicate an increasing trend in UAI in casual sexual encounters, from just over 20 per cent in 1999 to 38.3 per cent in 2012 and more recently a slight decline to 36.7 per cent in 2013 (Van de Ven et al., 2003; de Wit et al., 2014). The increase occurred across all states in Australia, including New South Wales, which suffered a 24 per cent increase in HIV diagnoses in 2012 when compared with 2011, followed by a decline in 2013 of 13 per cent when compared with 2012 (Gale et al., 2014). Also alarming is that this upward trend is more marked in men under 25 years of age. In 2012 HIV-positive men were increasingly more likely to disclose their status in casual encounters than they were a decade prior and, of the HIV-positive men on treatment, 90 per cent reported an undetectable viral load. Furthermore, the upward trend in UAIC was more marked among HIV-positive men than among HIV-negative men. This increase is disquieting for, as Zablotska et al. (2010) have demonstrated, declines in condom use among gay and other homosexually active men are associated with increases in HIV incidence in the same population.

These trends in the sexual behaviour of gay men in Australia, alongside rises in HIV incidence, suggest the importance of acknowledging and navigating the chasm between promising models of ideal TasP scenarios and real world conditions wherein elements of TasP may be partially in place or deployed in less than ideal ways. Understanding and addressing how elements of TasP are being taken up is vital before its promises can be embraced.

Conclusions

The contributing factors to Australia's early and relatively sustained success cannot be attributed to a single 'magic bullet' with which to respond to HIV. Rather, it can be attributed to what is known in Australia as 'the partnership': a partnership that is community engaged, politically active and provided with resources (Brown et al., 2014). Such a partnership – across community organisations, health services and clinicians, government health departments, political activists, researchers – is not easy to maintain. Partnerships are not static and, from 1997 to 1998, Australia witnessed disinvestment and political neglect in some states.

The approach taken in Australia that appeared to have been successful was the production of a 'social vaccine'. There were not widespread interventions by HIV-prevention scientists, behaviour-change experts and other specialists in the form of community-intervention trials. That 'industry' has simply not developed in Australia. In its place there has been a more broad-based and collective response. Community activism among gay men, as well as among other groups and communities – Indigenous communities, among people who inject drugs and among sex workers – has led the way, in dialogue with policymakers and enlightened politicians and in partnership with researchers in national and more local centres. As a result, affected communities have, in their own way come to 'own' the epidemic and worked toward engaging their constituent members as part of a coherent response. Prevention programmes in Australia have never been based on evidence of efficacy derived from randomised controlled trials, but on demonstrated effectiveness on the ground and in the belief that such an approach is, quite simply, the right thing to do.

Put slightly more theoretically, in the Australian response to HIV we can see clear evidence of what might be termed a 'social' public health, in which there has been (a) a focus on understanding and engaging *collectives* rather than the individual; (b) a focus on *social practice* and the structures or 'social drivers' that give rise to practice, rather than on individual behaviour; (c) a reliance on *grass-roots expertise* alongside medical, epidemiological and social research insights in the development of a widely owned health promotion approach; and (d) the adoption of a *tripartite approach* in which governments have worked together with communities and social and public health researchers to develop an effective, yet malleable, response (Kippax et al., 2013). Within social public health, prevention programmes or interventions are focused on resourcing communities or groups, not only to educate and teach skills to their constituent members about changing normative understandings and expectations, but also to act on their own behalf to advocate for change. HIV-prevention programmes provide support for social movements, and this emphasis on social change means that prevention approaches are understood as being in need of constant development so that they are relevant to the social practices that communities are devising and deploying now.

However, as in Uganda, in Australia today there is mounting evidence that the safe-sex culture that was produced in gay communities in response to the early crisis of HIV, is faltering. Research suggests this is in part a response to the fact that HIV is now a chronic disease. The evidence also indicates that the increasing medicalisation of prevention and the associated focus on testing and treatment for both HIV-negative as well as HIV-positive men may have also played a role in the faltering of the early successful response. We take up this issue of the medicalisation of prevention in the chapters that follow.

Part II

SOCIAL TRANSFORMATION

Chapter 4

THE BIOMEDICAL NARRATIVE
OF HIV/AIDS

The faltering of HIV/AIDS prevention – in some cases after initial successes as described in the two previous chapters – is cause for concern. Such concern may account for the embrace by many in biomedicine of advances such as male circumcision, pre-exposure prophylaxis (PrEP) and treatment as prevention (TasP). We believe this embrace to be premature and may, as we have suggested, exacerbate the 'faltering'. Although male circumcision is likely to help in reducing HIV transmission in generalised epidemics such as those in sub-Saharan Africa, it does not provide a complete solution. Furthermore, given the inconsistent results in regard to the efficacy of PrEP, and that evidence for the efficacy of TasP rests on studies of cohabiting couples, the calls for PrEP and TasP to be rolled out as major prevention initiatives for entire populations are troubling. Not only are there questions with regard to the efficacy of these prevention strategies, but there is confusion as to how public health would ensure their effectiveness.

Consider how Montaner spoke about TasP in an interview conducted during the 2013 International AIDS Society Conference on HIV Pathogenesis, Treatment and Prevention (IAS) Conference; an interview that occurred when TasP was endorsed by the World Health Organization (WHO) and included in its guidelines for HIV treatment and prevention (WHO, 2013b). Montaner argued: 'From a normative perspective we [proponents of TasP] are there. The next step is we need to recruit [...] [people] to do the very difficult work of implementation science [; ...] we want you to help us deliver under the promise of Treatment as Prevention'. The framing of TasP as heralding the 'end of AIDS' makes sense when we think of 'implementation science', as Montaner suggests – that is, simply (and simplistically) as enabling public health to ensure that people will do what public health deems best: if HIV-negative, test frequently and regularly for HIV and, if HIV-positive, take up and adhere to antiretroviral treatments (ART). However, as we have documented in the cases of Uganda and Australia and will further demonstrate in the remainder of this book, effective HIV prevention does not work like that.

Rather, it involves communication, especially talk, between people and within communities, talk that gives rise to efforts to develop social practices to adopt, rework or reject particular techniques of prevention – be they drugs, clean needles, condoms or negotiated agreements between sexual partners about risk-taking and risk-reduction. 'Implementation' is a misnomer that clouds the fact that any HIV-prevention strategy works (or not) to the extent it is adopted (and adapted) and made part of a community's social practices. That is, HIV-prevention strategies are inherently social, and the social worlds in which they operate cannot be reduced to 'implementation'. Whether prevention strategies are deemed biomedical or behavioural, this kind of attempt to sideline the social aspects of HIV and HIV prevention (as though those aspects matter only as 'enablers of' or 'barriers to' HIV transmission and prevention) is not unique to discussions of TasP – instead, it is a longstanding and confounding factor in the global response to HIV.

In this chapter we first describe how the social is rendered inexpressible by the biomedical narrative of HIV, and we illustrate this sidelining of the social in the Timeline of important events in the history of HIV produced by the Joint United Nations Programme on HIV/AIDS (UNAIDS). We then consider some of the mechanisms through which the social is continually portrayed as tangential to HIV prevention. In particular we examine two conceptual distinctions that serve to confuse rather than clarify. With regard to the first of these, we argue that the distinction biomedicine makes between HIV-prevention strategies in terms of whether they are behavioural or biomedical is incorrect (with the latter understood to employ 'technologies'). In the second case, we examine the distinction between efficacy and effectiveness of HIV-prevention strategies and discuss the very commonplace mishandling of this distinction by biomedical scientists. Although the concepts of efficacy and effectiveness are central to biomedicine, the biomedical narrative of HIV prevention appears far more concerned with efficacy than effectiveness. This privileging of efficacy serves to sideline the social aspects of HIV prevention, but more than this, it positions the social as a *barrier* to translating efficacious strategies into effective ones. We argue that this confusion over what is or is not an efficacious or effective prevention strategy (or 'technology') bolsters the biomedical narrative of HIV prevention, making understanding of the social practices pertaining to HIV prevention harder and harder to reach.

Inexpressibility of the Social

HIV is a social disease: it is transmitted by sexual practices and drug injection practices, both profoundly social activities. Although, as outlined in the preceding chapters, governments, communities and individuals have responded to reduce HIV incidence, many, indeed most, of the HIV-prevention or risk-reduction strategies that arose were of community. These strategies emerged out of people's social relations and their connections to one another via sex and other shared activities, and via sociability and talk. In Uganda and Australia and many other countries, they were adopted by members of communities at risk before public health endorsed their use. Nonetheless, as we demonstrate in this chapter, the history of HIV prevention as it has been told and continues to be told has an increasingly dominant biomedical inflection.

Although HIV treatment falls largely within the domain of biomedicine, HIV prevention sits across the domains of social science and biomedicine. Yet, viewing the global response to HIV from the perspective of South Africa, Fassin argues that, 'Since the beginning of the pandemic, the focus of discourse and policies throughout the world solely on the medical aspects of the illness, and since the beginning of the South African controversy, solely on the availability of drugs, has made the social issues (both carried and revealed by AIDS) practically inexpressible' (2007, 189). In this and the next two chapters we focus on the challenges of 'practically expressing' the social and of crossing what Adam (2011) calls the 'epistemic fault line' that has problematically opposed the social and biomedical sciences. The major challenge is to 'practically express the social' in an HIV/AIDS environment dominated by biomedicine. Effective prevention depends on crossing the fault line and expressing the social.

From the outset of the response to HIV, the biomedical narrative has always been the dominant one. Initially, the biomedical narrative was primarily concerned with diagnosis, HIV testing and treatment, and the search for a vaccine. The social narrative was concerned, in the main, with prevention and the social, cultural and political factors associated with HIV transmission and the impact of HIV on people and societies. Notwithstanding UNAIDS position papers such as Intensifying HIV Prevention (UNAIDS, 2005), since 1996, with the advent of successful treatments for HIV, the biomedical voice has become more dominant.

UNAIDS Timeline

This dominance is clearly illustrated in the UNAIDS Timeline of HIV published in 2006 (see Table 4.1) representing the important events in the HIV/AIDS history (UNAIDS, 2006). The history begins in June 1981 with the diagnosis of a devastating immune deficiency disease in a young gay man in the United States. In 1982 the acquired immune deficiency disease (AIDS) was named and in 1983 HIV was identified as the cause of AIDS. Later in that same year in Africa, the heterosexual AIDS epidemic was acknowledged. A

Table 4.1 UNAIDS Timeline.

1981	Young gay man 'diagnosed' with devastating immune deficiency in the United States
1982	Acquired immune deficiency syndrome (AIDS) named
1983	Human immunodeficiency virus (HIV) was identified as the cause of AIDS and the heterosexual epidemic revealed in Africa
1985	Test to detect HIV in infected persons with no symptoms developed – HIV test
1986	Global Network of People Living with HIV/AIDS (GNP+) founded
1987	Global Program on AIDS (World Health Organization) was established in recognition of a global epidemic
1987	First therapy for AIDS – AZT (zidovudine) – developed
1993	In 1991 to 1993, HIV prevalence in young pregnant women in Uganda and in young men in Thailand begins to decrease, the first major downturn in developing countries
1994	First treatment regimen to reduce mother-to-child transmission developed
1996	Comparatively successful antiretroviral treatment (ART) developed
1996	Joint United Nations Programme on HIV/AIDS (UNAIDS) formed
1997	Brazil becomes first developing country to provide ART through its public health system
2001	United Nations General Special Session on AIDS (UNGASS) is held in recognition of growing global concern
2001	Global Fund to Fight HIV, Tuberculosis, and Malaria established
2003	The 3 by 5 Initiative of the World Health Organization (3 million people on ART by 2005) developed
2004	Global Coalition on Women and AIDS launched

Source: Adapted from UNAIDS (2006, 4).*

couple of years later, in 1985, UNAIDS notes the development of a test to detect HIV infection in persons who show no signs of disease. The development and approval for use in the United States of the first therapy for HIV (AZT, zidovudine) came late in 1987. Although AZT did not prove to be a very effective treatment, its availability encouraged HIV testing and raised the hopes of those living with HIV. Up until that time there was no treatment for AIDS except palliative care of symptoms and associated infections.

After the first seven years there is a big gap, at least as portrayed by UNAIDS (UNAIDS, 2006). Then in 1993 the decline in HIV prevalence in Uganda (among pregnant women) and Thailand (among young men) is noted, and in 1994 the UNAIDS Timeline notes the development of the first treatment regimen to reduce transmission from mother to child – later called the prevention of mother-to-child transmission (PMTCT). And in 1996, 15 years after the inkling of something amiss in 1981, biomedicine developed the first really effective treatment –ART – not a cure but an effective therapy that meant that AIDS was held at bay and, for most people on treatment, HIV became a chronic illness. The first effective treatments for those living with HIV, ART and the associated move to roll out HIV testing is a watershed in the history of the HIV/AIDS epidemic. A year later, in 1997, Brazil made ART available to all its citizens through its public health system – the first middle-income country to do so.

Alongside these developments in biomedicine, the UNAIDS Timeline also notes that there were political developments. In 1986 the Global Network of People Living with HIV/AIDS (GNP+), then the International Steering Committee of People Living with HIV/AIDS, was founded, and this was followed in mid-1987 by the launching of WHO's Global Programme on AIDS – in recognition of the scale of the problem. In the same year as ART was made available, UNAIDS was formed to organise and coordinate the work of a number of UN agencies – UNESCO, UNDP, and so forth. Then 2001 was marked by a meeting of the United Nations General Special Session (UNGASS) – with worldwide acknowledgment of the severity of the problem and of how the vulnerability of particular population groups to HIV infection demanded recognition as a security issue. Also that year was the establishment of The Global Fund to Fight AIDS, TB and Malaria, a public–private international financing organisation launched in January 2002. In 2003 we see the development of the 3X5 initiative of WHO and UNAIDS with the aim of reaching 3 million people in the developing world with ART by 2005. And although not included in the original UNAIDS Timeline, as noted in Chapter 2 in the same year, President George W. Bush committed $15 billion over five years (2003–2008) in the scheme called the President's Emergency Plan for AIDS Relief (PEPFAR) to fight HIV, with most of the funding devoted to treatment. The final note on the UNAIDS historical timeline is the formation of the Global Coalition on Women and AIDS in 2004.

Updated timeline: Biomedical prevention strategies

The UNAIDS Timeline has a decidedly biomedical refrain and privileges treatment over prevention (see Table 4.1). The major moments in the timeline are indisputably the development of the HIV test (1985) and the development of successful ART (1996). And although in 1984 US Health and Human Services secretary, Margaret Heckler, optimistically predicted there would be an AIDS vaccine ready for testing by 1986, the search for an effective vaccine and for a cure continues. Prevention was referred to only twice: once in 1993 in terms of declines in HIV in Uganda and Thailand and there was no mention of how such declines occurred; and in 1994 in terms of the use of treatment regimens to reduce mother-to-child transmission.

Since the UNAIDS Timeline was published, the biomedical narrative has become more dominant and is increasingly focused on the development of HIV-prevention strategies, typically referred to as biomedical prevention technologies or tools: male circumcision, the use of ART for prevention – as in PrEP, post-exposure prophylaxis (PEP) and microbicides – and the use of ART as prevention (TasP), as shown in our extension of the UNAIDS Timeline below (see Table 4.2).

All of these, with the exception of male circumcision, which has been shown to be moderately efficacious (around 60%) in preventing the sexual transmission of HIV from women to men (Auvert et al., 2005; Gray et al., 2007; Bailey et al., 2007), are based on the use of various forms of ART in prevention. These strategies are PrEP, in the form of oral ART, which has been shown to be efficacious in reducing the risk of HIV transmission among men engaging in anal intercourse (Grant et al., 2010[1]) but has had very mixed results when trialled with heterosexuals (Baeten et al., 2012[2]; Van Damme et al., 2012[3]; Thigpen et al., 2012[4]; ongoing VOICE study[5]); microbicides in the form of a vaginal gel, which have shown low efficacy for preventing HIV infection in women (Abdool, et al., 2010[6]); and PEP which, if used within 72 hours of HIV exposure, has a proven track record for occupational exposure (Cardo et al., 1997) and has been adopted in some countries for non-occupational exposure, for example in Australia (ANCAHRD, 2001). These prevention strategies are primarily intended for those who are HIV-negative or have had

Table 4.2 Updated UNAIDS Timeline: 2005–2014.

2005, 2007	Male circumcision found to be moderately efficacious in reducing the risk of transmission from women to men
2008	Reauthorisation of PEPFAR and development of bilaterally funded programmes
2008	Swiss Consensus Statement (treatment as prevention, TasP): Observational data demonstrate that for serodiscordant cohabiting heterosexual couples, by lowering the viral load to undetectable levels, ART reduces risk of infection of the HIV-negative partner by 96%
2010	Low efficacy demonstrated for microbicide vaginal gel
2010, 2012	Mixed results re efficacy of pre-exposure prophylaxis in oral form
2012, 2014	Randomised controlled trials (RCTs) confirm the efficacy of TasP for both heterosexual and homosexual cohabiting serodiscordant couples
2013	WHO Guidelines on the use of ART for treating and prevention HIV
2014	CDC Guideline on use of PrEP in the USA

a recent exposure to HIV. More recently, as discussed earlier, there has been a push to provide ART to all people living with HIV so as to lower their infectivity and so reduce the population viral load. This prevention strategy – referred to as 'treatment as prevention (TasP)' or 'test and treat' (Granich et al., 2009; Cohen et al., 2012; Rodger et al., 2014) – is manifest in the WHO's (2013b) guidelines.

Biomedical experts and researchers are not the only ones privileging biomedical solutions: AVAC, the Global Advocacy for HIV Prevention nongovernmental organisation, lists only PrEP, microbicides, vaccines, and TasP in a 2013 website update on prevention (http://data.avac.org/WorldMap.aspx). Yet the timing of the initial HIV-prevention successes in Uganda and Australia, as described in Chapters 2 and 3, and in a range of other countries, referred to in Chapter 1, and the global decline of HIV incidence, indicates that none of these early successes can be attributed to the so-called biomedical prevention technologies – unless one includes condoms as a biomedical intervention. So what is going on? We believe that the answer to this question has to do with the ways in which biomedicine understands prevention and in the ways in which it understands evidence. We discuss this by turning to ill-conceived efforts to categorise prevention strategies and to find evidence for their impact. But, first, we discuss what is involved in HIV prevention.

HIV-Prevention Strategies and Social Practice

There are a large number of HIV-prevention strategies that have been, and continue to be, used – some more efficacious than others, some effective in some contexts but less so in others and some whose efficacy or effectiveness has yet to be established. There are also strategies employed by governments to ensure that the blood supply is secure, and there is the PMTCT strategy. Here, however, we focus on HIV transmission and its prevention in relation to engaging in sexual intercourse and injecting drugs.

Some HIV-prevention strategies to avoid or reduce the risk of *sexual* transmission of HIV are:

- the delaying of the initiation of sexual intercourse or, in a more extreme form, abstinence from sexual intercourse;
- reduction of the number of partners with whom one engages in sexual intercourse or, in a more extreme form, monogamy;
- condom use – both male and female condoms;
- withdrawal before ejaculation during sexual intercourse;
- male circumcision;

- serosorting: engaging in sexual intercourse with someone whose serostatus is known or assumed to be the same as one's own, including the special case of negotiated safety (as described in Chapter 3);
- strategic positioning: a strategy that can be used by gay and other homosexually active men in which the HIV-negative partner is the insertive partner and the HIV-positive partner is receptive;
- anti-retroviral treatments (ART) – for use by HIV-negative persons – in the form of microbicide gels or oral drugs as in pre-exposure prophylaxis (PrEP) and post-exposure prophylaxis (PEP);
- ART – for use by HIV-positive persons – to lower their viral load to undetectable levels to protect their cohabiting HIV-negative partners.

For those who inject drugs, prevention strategies include:

- abstinence (which is often enabled by the use of non-injectable opioid drugs such as methadone);
- use of sterile needles and syringes;
- anti-retroviral treatments (ART) – for use by HV-negative persons – in the form of oral drugs as in pre-exposure prophylaxis (PrEP) or post-exposure prophylaxis (PEP).

There are important differences between these strategies from the point of view of the people who, if they have access, might adopt one or more of them. With the exception of male circumcision and, to a lesser extent, PEP, all current prevention strategies need to be invoked over and over again and built into people's everyday lives. Their sustained use is extremely difficult, if not impossible, unless they are incorporated into everyday practices. Prevention strategies differ with reference to whether they are intimately tied to sexual practices, drug injecting activity and people's daily routines. Sterile needles and syringes must be incorporated into the act of injecting and are unlikely to be effective unless people can make them part of their injecting practice. Condoms demand that people negotiate the introduction of their use into their sexual practices and, although the use of microbicide gels does not demand negotiation, their use is closely linked to sexual practice. Similarly, although they are somewhat less physically intrusive than condom use, strategies such as abstinence and serosorting are also tied to people's sexual practices: for example, abstinence is not simply a decision, it has to be enacted. TasP and PrEP differ again in that medication needs to be interwoven into another set of practices involving the minutiae of daily routines of eating and sleeping as well as regular medical consultations for monitoring. These differences clearly have an impact on how strategies are taken up and their use sustained, that is, their long-term effectiveness in reducing HIV incidence. There is little doubt, for example, that taking a pill as in PrEP – if it is affordable, side-effect free and involves a relatively manageable regimen – could be much easier for many than using a condom. On the other hand, if one is an HIV-negative sex-worker, the promotion of PrEP as HIV prevention is likely to be seen as undermining working practices that involve clients' use of condoms: PrEP might be unacceptable to sex workers on the grounds that its use exposes them to sexually transmissible infections other than HIV, and to the potential long-term side effects of PrEP. In general, differentiating prevention strategies according to the social practices involved in their effective use is useful, as it prompts consideration of those social practices and of the challenges for people, communities and public health institutions that are trying to build on or initiate shifts in practice.

Biomedicine and Its Understanding of Prevention

Biomedicine does not distinguish between the many HIV-prevention strategies in the above manner. Rather, biomedicine regards some HIV-prevention strategies as behavioural and others as biomedical in the sense that they are dependent on the use of drugs or other technologies or tools. Such a distinction has clouded efforts to identify and understand the effectiveness of distinct strategies for particular contexts.

Under the rubric of strategies premised on technologies we commonly find ART in its various prevention forms and male circumcision, as well as those strategies involving the use of sterile needles and syringes and condoms – although it is of interest to note that these last-mentioned strategies initially emerged from affected communities of gay men and networks of people who inject drugs and not from biomedicine.[7] These technologies are promoted as part of HIV-prevention interventions or HIV-prevention programmes, which biomedical professionals largely view as the work of 'implementation scientists'. Framed this way, when efficacious technologies are implemented without good results, the problem can appear to be their implementation, and the vital need to understand their effectiveness in real-world contexts is glossed over. Furthermore, the use of the terms *technologies* or *tools* places abstinence, reduction of number of partners, as well as a number of other so-called behavioural HIV-prevention strategies such as negotiated safety, serosorting, strategic positioning, and so forth in a very odd space (or non-space, the non-space we have indicated by their absence in our extension of the UNAIDS Timeline, see Table 4.2 above).

The value of distinguishing technology-based strategies from behavioural strategies is highly questionable, as all prevention strategies – whether they involve the use of a tool or technology – require some change in behaviour or, rather, *practice*, in the sense that sexual and drug injection practices and dosing practices are organised and patterned by culture and regulated by social norms (Kippax, 2008). Such norms enable and regulate the ways in which people take medicine such as PrEP, or use condoms for sexual activity, adopt male circumcision, reduce the numbers of their sexual partners, disclose their HIV status to sexual partners or infer and make decisions about HIV status and infectivity of their potential partners. It quickly becomes a meaningless distinction: negotiated safety, for example, is behavioural in that it requires people who are having sex with each other to change their practices, to test, to discuss test results, to discuss sex outside of the relationship and possibly to dispense with condoms where they have been used to date. But it is also clearly involves a technology: without the technology of the HIV test, and without an informed group of people who understand some of the intricacies of testing and results, the behavioural changes would be meaningless. Similarly, 'strategic positioning' relies on an understanding (real or imagined) of the insertive sexual partner's HIV status. At the same time, as we indicated above, most strategies deemed 'technologised' require sustained changes in practice: clean needles have to be accessed and used each time a person injects; condoms have to be accessed and used every time one has sex; PrEP needs to be taken according to a strict regimen in order to be effective, so unless they are incorporated into social practices, they will be useless or worse; and so on.

So what is the point of repeatedly designating a prevention strategy as involving a technology or otherwise? The value (to some) we argue is that it serves to shore up a misleading distinction between biomedical and behavioural strategies, with biomedical ones involving technologies. The problem with the behavioural–biomedical distinction is that strategies that appear clearly behavioural, like strategic positioning, require – are premised on – people's engagement with biomedicine. Likewise a biomedical strategy entailing ART requires the sustained incorporation of drugs or microbicide gels into people's everyday lives – that is, changes to their social practices. Whether these strategies are deemed biomedical technologies or not is, to a large degree, irrelevant. All prevention strategies, including those that are sometimes called biomedical and those that are technology-based, are to a greater or lesser extent socially and culturally produced and imbued with meaning.

In failing to acknowledge the ways in which prevention strategies differ from one another according to the specific practices entailed in their adoption, in failing to recognise that all prevention strategies require changes in the social practices of people, and in claiming ownership of so called biomedical technologies, biomedicine erases the social. Prevention becomes something that public health workers offer to, or 'do' to, individuals. The fact that people are social beings – members of communities and networks in which they have sex and inject drugs – goes unrecognised and unacknowledged, or is cast, as Montaner does in his vision of the future of TaSP, as belonging to the terrain of 'implementation science'.[8]

Biomedicine and Its Understanding of Evidence

Another reason that biomedicine has difficulty with HIV prevention is related to how it assesses evidence in relation to safety, efficacy and effectiveness. Safety in terms of the toxicity of drugs is generally assessed early in the development of treatments and prophylactic drugs and will not be addressed in detail here: our major concern is in regard to efficacy and effectiveness, although safety in terms of the impact of new strategies on current HIV-prevention strategies will be addressed.

Public health's role is to ensure the safety, efficacy and effectiveness of HIV-prevention strategies – those that public health promotes, and those that people have produced themselves, such as condom use and serosorting. It is important to know whether strategies are safe and that they 'work', that is, whether they result in the sustained reduction of HIV transmission in the population. However, biomedicine appears to privilege efficacy, in that once safety (in the sense of non-toxicity) is assured and efficacy demonstrated, the prevention strategy (e.g., TasP) is widely promoted in the absence of monitoring of long-term effectiveness at the population level or without knowledge of its effectiveness in specific contexts.

Efficacy

Efficacy is generally accepted to be 'the improvement in health outcome, achieved in a research setting, in expert hands, under ideal circumstances' (Aral & Peterman, 1999, 33). Typically, efficacy is assessed under controlled experimental conditions and, in particular, in a randomised controlled trial (RCT). Over the last few years, it has been shown that the following strategies are safe and that they are efficacious – at least to some degree (see Table 4.3).

All the above have been subject to one or more randomised trials. In the case of condoms, tested via simulated use, the findings indicate that both male and female condoms are highly efficacious, although male condoms have a slightly higher efficacy. Male circumcision, which reduces HIV transmission from women to men, has been found to be moderately efficacious. The strategies based on ART have a wider range of efficacy. The prevention of mother-to-child transmission (PMTCT) has been shown to have high efficacy, microbicides to have low efficacy in preventing HIV infection

Table 4.3 Efficacy of HIV-prevention strategies established by experiment.

Strategy	Efficacy
Male Condoms	95% (Van De Perre et al., 1987; Carey et al., 1992).
Female Condoms	90–95% (Minnis & Padian, 2005)
PMTCT	High efficacy dependent on drug regimen (Leroy et al. (2002); Lallemant et al. (2004).
Vaginal Microbicides	39% (Abdool Karim et al., 2010)
Pre-exposure Prophylaxis (PrEP)	Range from 0% to 63% to 92% (Grant et al., 2010; Baeten et al., 2012; Van Damme et al., 2012; and Thigpen et al., 2012)
Treatment as Prevention (TasP)	96% (Cohen et al., 2012; Rodger et al., 2014)
Male Circumcision	58% (Auvert et al., 2005; Gray et al., 2007; Bailey et al., 2007).

among women (Abdool et al., 2010), and the results with regard to PrEP are mixed. Grant et al. (2010), in a six-country study, found that on average PrEP (once-daily TDF/FTC) reduced HIV transmission among gay men and other men who have sex with men by 44 per cent, although among those men who had a high dosing adherence, efficacy rose to 92 per cent. In other randomised controlled studies among heterosexuals in Kenya (Baeten et al., 2012), efficacy was calculated at 73 per cent, while in Botswana (Thigpen et al., 2012) it was 63 per cent. However in 2011 a study among women was stopped because of an ongoing lack of significance between the placebo and experimental arms of the study (Van Damme et al., 2012). Further studies evaluating PrEP are ongoing. The strategy of treating those infected with HIV as soon after infection as possible (TasP) has been shown to be highly efficacious, 96 per cent, for heterosexual cohabiting couples living in sero-discordant relationships (Cohen et al., 2012) and for male couples, likewise (Rodger et al., 2014).

There are some HIV-prevention strategies the efficacy of which need not be established under experimental conditions. There is no need for RCTs with regard to abstinence and the use of sterile needles and syringes: logically, absti-nence is 100 per cent efficacious, as is the use of sterile needles and syringes. If a person does not engage in sexual intercourse at all, then they will not be infected with HIV via sexual transmission; and a person who injects drugs cannot be infected if she/he uses sterile needles and syringes[9] (see Table 4.4).

The efficacy of the following HIV-prevention strategies is difficult to evaluate: delaying sexual initiation and reduction in number of partners are likely to reduce the sexual transmission of HIV in any given population,

Table 4.4 Efficacy of HIV-prevention strategies established without experiment.

Strategy	Efficacy
Abstinence	100%
Sterile Needles and Syringes	100%
Reduction in Number of Sexual/Drug Injection Partners	Dependent on number and HIV status of partners
Serosorting	100% if apprised of correct information, and sexual partners are concordant for HIV: either both HIV-negative or HIV-positive
Strategic positioning	Insertive sex less risky than receptive sex, but efficacy unknown
Post-exposure Prophylaxis (PEP)	81% (Cardo et al., 1997)
Withdrawal	Unknown

and although serial monogamy may reduce HIV in the population, fidelity will protect HIV-negative persons if and only if their sexual partners are also HIV-negative and do not engage in unprotected sex outside their relationship. Serosorting is by definition 100 per cent efficacious, at least in the case of negative–negative sex or positive–positive sex. The efficacy of strategic positioning is unknown, and although it is known that receptive sex places one at greater risk of HIV than insertive sex, insertive sex also carries risk of HIV-transmission. An RCT in the case of PEP is considered unethical, however, for those who take up the post-exposure drugs in the form of ART within 36 hours of potential exposure to HIV and adhere to the drug regimen, the data demonstrate an efficacy of around 81 per cent (see Table 4.4).

Although many of these strategies are efficacious, only some of them have been promoted by public health: abstinence and delaying sexual initiation and the reduction of number of sexual partners – as the AB – of the ABC of prevention, and – in almost all countries – condom use. Although serosorting in some form (for example, unprotected sex between two HIV-negative or HIV-positive people) cannot transmit HIV, it has not generally been promoted. The exceptions are to be found in Australia and to some degree the Netherlands and Malaysia, albeit in somewhat different ways. In Australia, as discussed in Chapter 3, a form of serosorting, 'negotiated safety' was promoted between seroconcordant HIV-negative couples (Kinder, 1996) and later in the Netherlands (Davidovich et al., 2000). In Malaysia, in the Muslim population mandatory HIV testing was introduced for couples planning marriage (Burns, 2009).

Effectiveness

The effectiveness of strategies – whether they involve the use of so-called tech-nologies or changes in practices such as partner-reduction – is largely depen-dent on whether they are taken up and adhered to and also whether their use disrupts other HIV-prevention strategies. Their effectiveness is dependent on social and cultural factors. Although it is comparatively straightforward to demonstrate efficacy, it is far more complex to show that any given prevention strategy is effective.

Effectiveness is defined as 'the impact an intervention achieves in the real world, under resource constraints, in entire populations or specified sub-groups of a population. It is the improvement in health outcome' (Aral & Peterman, 1999, 33). In order to ensure effectiveness, social changes or changes in prac-tice are needed because, broadly stated, every HIV-prevention strategy has one or more associated behavioural components that can influence its success or failure. Without changes in practice, there is little likelihood of widespread adoption and sustained use of HIV-prevention strategies. For each HIV-prevention strategy, what is needed are data that indicate whether it is socially and culturally acceptable, whether it has been taken up/adopted and whether its use has been sustained over time. That is, what is needed are data demon-strating effectiveness. While efficacy is necessary to lower HIV incidence in populations, it is not sufficient. Effectiveness of any of these strategies depends on their uptake in the real world under real-world conditions such as acces-sibility, socio-cultural acceptance and sustainability, and political acceptance (see Table 4.5 below).

As Kippax (2003) has argued, the assessment of effectiveness is a local and particular matter. Designed to isolate and identify cause and effect, RCTs are, in general, inappropriate to measure or assess effectiveness: it is highly unlikely that there is any simple causal relationship between any given HIV-prevention strategy advocated and HIV incidence, at least in the short term. Further-more, while it is claimed that it is 'the intervention' that is being evaluated in an RCT purporting to assess effectiveness, there is often confusion in these studies over whether it is the prevention strategy or technology or its mode of promotion that is being evaluated. In other words, there is often confusion between the 'medium', that is, the manner in which the prevention technology or strategy is promoted – counselling, school education, peer education, and so forth, and the 'message', that is the technology or prevention tool that is being promoted – condoms, circumcision, and so forth. For example, counsel-ling and testing are very often inappropriately placed in the same category as condoms: the former is a means of promoting the use of the latter.

Effectiveness is contingent on a large number of variables, including those shown in Table 4.5, as well as on the efficacy of the prevention strategy or

Table 4.5 Effectiveness of HIV-prevention strategies.

Prevention Strategy	Cost	Social Acceptance	Political Acceptability	Effectiveness
Abstinence/ Delayed sexual activity	None	Dependent on particular population	Acceptable	Effective in some few populations but generally ineffective over long term
Reduction in number of partners	None	Dependent on particular population	Acceptable	Effective in some populations
Serosorting	Cost of HIV Test	Acceptable	Acceptable in some countries	Effective under special conditions, otherwise unknown
Sterile Needles & Syringes	Low	Acceptable by those who inject drugs	Acceptable in some countries	Effective in countries where supplied
Male Condoms	Low	Acceptable to many but not all	Acceptable	Effective in some populations
Female Condoms	Relatively low	Acceptable to many but not all	Acceptable	Effective in some populations
PMTCT	Medium	Acceptable	Acceptable	Effective
Microbicides	Medium to high	Acceptable	Acceptable	Ineffective because of low efficacy
PrEP	High cost	Acceptable to some	Mixed response	Unknown
PEP	Medium	Acceptable	Mixed response	Where available, moderately effective
TasP	High	Acceptable to some	Acceptable	Effective under special conditions (i.e., monogamous cohabiting couples)
Male Circumcision	Medium	Acceptable to some but not others	Acceptable in some countries not others	Moderately effective for heterosexual men

technology. Methods that enable the long-term monitoring of the reception, adoption and sustained use of the HIV-prevention strategies that have been promoted are needed in order to evaluate effectiveness: biomedicine refers to these studies as Phase IV studies. Such evidence of effectiveness has been made available via HIV-incidence figures and behavioural surveillance data that are now collected in many countries and where these can be linked to the HIV-prevention strategies that were in play over time. For example, valid evidence in the form of both retrospective and ongoing monitoring studies, as well as rich, 'thick' descriptions of social processes, can be and has been provided for HIV-prevention strategies in Uganda (see Chapter 2), Australia (see Chapter 3), Thailand (Hanenberg et al., 1994) and Switzerland (Dubois-Arber et al., 1993; Dubois-Arber et al., 1999; Dubois-Arber et al., 2003). In a series of reports, The Global HIV Prevention Working Group (2002, 2003, 2004, 2006, 2007, 2008) documents many prevention successes. Also of particular note are studies that have used modelling as well as the monitoring of HIV incidence and behavioural surveillance in particular populations, in conjunction with describing the country's response, including its prevention programmes. These studies have identified the factors historically connected with the uptake of the prevention strategies associated with changes in practice and changes in HIV incidence. The better the data – the social, including ethnographic data, as well as the surveillance data – the more accurate is the assessment of effectiveness. Such evidence has been provided for Uganda by Hallett et al. (2006), and for Zimbabwe by Hallett et al. (2006), Gregson et al. (2006) and Halperin et al. (2011). Data such as these enable researchers to identify the key factors associated with declining HIV-transmission rates in specific contexts.

On the basis of findings from studies such as those described above, we have evidence for the effectiveness (or otherwise) of a range of HIV-prevention strategies. To date we know that the use of sterile needles and syringes, male and female condoms, PMTCT and PEP are effective in reducing HIV transmission in *most* populations. We also know that although abstinence is efficacious, it is not generally effective in reducing the sexual transmission of HIV, although delaying sexual initiation can be effective – for example, in Uganda in the 1980s (discussed in Chapter 2). With reference to gay men in Australia, the evidence indicates that with the exception of negotiated safety, a form of highly effective serosorting engaged in by regular sexual partners, serosorting with casual partners is at best only partially effective (Jin et al., 2009). In the same study, Jin et al. demonstrate that while strategic positioning is moderately effective, withdrawal is not. Studies (see Gray et al., 2012; Westercamp et al., 2014) evaluating the effectiveness of male circumcision have found it to be moderately effective in the southern African countries, where male circumcision has been promoted, and neither of these studies found any evidence for risk compensation. It has not as yet been shown that PrEP, in either microbicide gel form or as oral drugs, is effective – in the sense that adoption and sustained use have been achieved and that HIV incidence has declined over time in the populations where these strategies have been rolled out.

Although it is highly likely that TasP is effective in protecting the HIV-negative partner of a serodiscordant cohabiting couple under the special conditions outlined by Vernazza et al. (2008), the available evidence is inconsistent with regard to the effectiveness of TasP at the *population* level. A few studies show a decline in HIV incidence over time in association with widespread uptake of ART: in British Columbia, Canada, a decline in HIV acquisition was associated with the uptake of ART among people who inject drugs (Montaner et al., 2010)[10]; in San Francisco, results suggested that high ART coverage led to reduced HIV transmission (Das et al., 2010); and in KwaZulu-Natal, where increasing coverage of ART in a very large population-based prospective cohort study was associated with a decline in the risk of HIV acquisition in the surrounding local community (Tanser et al., 2013). However, with the above notable exceptions, as the number of people on ART has increased, in many communities and regions there has been *no* concomitant decline in HIV incidence in populations, for example in Australia, New Zealand, continental Europe (France and the Netherlands), the United Kingdom, and North America, in particular among gay communities (Saxton et al., 2011; Wilson, 2012). Indeed, in some of these countries there have been increases in HIV incidence, and some socio-behavioural studies in Australia and in France, for example, show that among HIV-positive gay men (and their partners) with undetectable viral load there are increased levels of unprotected anal intercourse (Zablotska et al., 2009; Bavington et al., 2013), indicating that TasP or the rhetoric around TasP may have disrupted or disinhibited the use of condoms. This issue is discussed in detail in Chapter 7.

Much of the above evidence showing effectiveness or the lack of it appears to be ignored in biomedicine. In part, we believe, because efficacy is what is deemed important in biomedicine and, in part, because the evidence relating to effectiveness is not based on the outcome of RCTs or experiments and, hence, is mistakenly rejected by many in biomedicine (Padian et al., 2010). Effectiveness is local and particular – it is contingent. And this contingency challenges the understanding of the RCT as the gold standard of knowledge about HIV prevention: RCTs are designed to avoid the 'confounding' effects of local and particular contexts and practices, rather than to interrogate them. Insisting on RCTs to assess effectiveness has had very negative outcomes: most RCTs attempting to assess the 'effectiveness' of HIV prevention have reported 'non-significant' results. This leads to conclusions, framed within biomedical ways of thinking that HIV-prevention strategies are not working. It is a mistake to forego external validity for the sake of experimental precision. Social transformation is not amenable to experiment because effectiveness is the *contingent* outcome of the collective activity of a diverse range of actors, both human and non-human, including the prevention strategies themselves, scientific practices, clinical services, cultural, political and social environments, and the norms, values and discourses that animate human behaviour or practice (Race, 2012). There is evidence for prevention effectiveness, but the evidence is 'soft' and is highly likely to vary from place to place, from population to population. Over time, we need more of it – prospective cohorts, snapshots and real-world data.

In general, in biomedicine there is a glossing-over of the difference between efficacy and effectiveness, and there is a sense that many in biomedicine believe that 'patients' or individuals who are targeted by 'interventions' will simply do as requested by their doctors and adopt the strategies that have been demonstrated to be efficacious: good 'implementation' is all that is needed. Notwithstanding 'implementation science', many people will not do as required or suggested, whether that entails using a condom or adhering to a drug regimen or being tested frequently for HIV. More importantly, people are subject to many messages about safety and risk – and not only from public health. A decline in HIV incidence is not merely a matter of changing individuals' behaviours, but supporting and enabling populations and networks of individuals, communities, to transform their social practices in ways that make sense to them – at least until an effective prophylactic vaccine is produced and made available to all.

The bio-technologising, or biomedical move, while central to the fight against HIV and AIDS, has led to a downplaying of the role of social and cultural factors in the prevention of HIV: the social becomes positioned as a barrier to the effectiveness of efficacious prevention strategies – a problem for 'implementation scientists', and this is especially true in the case of some of the newer strategies. However, what is clear is that particular prevention strategies are acceptable to particular populations – but not to all, and to particular governments – but not to all. For example, although male circumcision is efficacious to the extent that it reduces the sexual transmission of HIV from women to men by 58 per cent, its effectiveness among the Hindu population in India is likely to be close to zero as male circumcision is culturally unacceptable to Hindus. Similarly, while condoms may be used properly and consistently with casual sexual partners by some populations in some parts of the world, their use is less likely within stable relationships such as marriage or concurrent regular and committed relationships where assumptions of fidelity make it difficult. Furthermore, most HIV-prevention strategies need to be sustained over time. Social transformation and the embedding of preventive practices in everyday life are necessary to translate efficacious strategies into effective ones.

The 'faltering' of HIV prevention is in part a function of the unwillingness of biomedicine to accept that social transformation is difficult to predict and takes time. It is possible that this impatience and the increasing dominance of biomedicine may make prevention even more difficult to achieve. While Cleland & Watkins (2006), among others, suggest that despite massive expenditure, HIV prevention has achieved little, social scientists such as Stillwagon (2006) and Caceres & Race (2010) suggest that the global analysis has been based on flawed methods and analysis, and on the reluctance to address the social nature of sexual and drug-use practices.

Conclusions

The confusing distinction with regard to what is or is not a behavioural strategy or a biomedical technological strategy deflects attention away from the fact that the effectiveness of all efficacious HIV-prevention strategies relies to a greater or lesser extent on changes in practice and social transformation. Attending to social practices and to changes in practice is further deflected by the misunderstandings rife in biomedicine with regard to efficacy and effectiveness, and their conflation has led to a curious insistence on using randomised controlled trials as the gold standard of evidence for the impact of HIV strategies when RCTs are generally unable to show any effectiveness in preventing HIV transmission. Fetishising methods creates industrial-scale research, but such research risks neglecting the very object it is supposed to help us address: patterns in HIV transmission.

As we will detail in the next chapters, the HIV pandemic is driven not by the individual actions of risk-takers or vulnerable subjects. Rather, HIV is driven primarily by patterns of practice, patterns produced by social and cultural norms and expectations. This means that prevention strategies will be effective only inasmuch as the human and socio-cultural aspects of their uptake and sustained use are satisfactorily addressed. Recently, attention has moved *from* the social *to* the biological/technological realm – *from* effectiveness *to* efficacy. We need to redress the balance. As Michael Clatts noted over ten years ago with reference to the trajectory of HIV research:

> [T]he process has gone terribly awry, […] the undaunted search for quick-fix models forces us to crawl into very narrow boxes, […] it jeopardizes our ability to see the world as it is, as well as our ability to offer constructive ideas about how

to change it. In my experience such models inevitably end up trying to fit the subject to the technology, rather than the other way around. (Clatts, 1994, 95)

One of the unique contributions that social scientists can make is explaining how practices – such as male circumcision or condom use – are influenced by the specific historical moment and the socio-cultural conditions in which they are adopted and enacted. The explanations for the adoption of male circumcision as a common (or rare) practice, or the uptake and sustained use of condoms, are unlikely to come in the form of linear, causal relationships. Rather, they will involve understanding multiple and diverse socio-cultural factors involved in shaping *patterns* of practice and changes in those patterns that rely, in turn, on the acceptability, uptake and sustained use of a prevention strategy. Biological or, indeed, psychological processes are not the only processes shaping variations in human behaviour: the other major forces are social, cultural and historical. The evidence available suggests that declines in HIV follow changes in people's sexual and injecting practices – whether and how people's adoption of so-called biomedical prevention strategies will or will not be associated with further reductions in HIV transmission demands interrogation. But, more broadly, any understanding of HIV transmission and prevention needs to begin by navigating and countering the institutionalised approaches to prevention – in the form of terms such as biomedical or behavioural prevention, or elisions between efficacious and effective strategies – approaches that function to render 'the social issues (both carried and revealed by AIDS) practically inexpressible' (Fassin, 2007, 189).

Chapter 5

RISK AND VULNERABILITY

Reviewing the history of HIV as it is sketched in the Joint United Nations Programme on HIV/AIDS (UNAIDS) Timeline in a little more detail is instructive. The young men in the United States who were dying in 1981 and 1982 were dying of rare illnesses that typically, in earlier years, had been effectively dealt with by the immune system. Gay men, mostly well-educated and socially upwardly mobile men, were dying of an unusual form of pneumonia and developing unusual cancers. Some in biomedicine believed that the poor immune response was related in some way to these young men's lifestyles: hence, the naming of the syndrome as the gay-related immune deficiency response, or GRID, or more nastily, the 'gay plague'. Although identified later, at around the same time, large numbers of people who injected drugs were also affected by and began to die of the same illnesses. Their deaths were also attributed to a notion of 'poor immune response' and, by extension, their lifestyles.

In one sense, the concerned clinicians and biomedical scientists were correct: the observed patterns of illness and the deaths were an indirect result of a poor immune system and the 'poor immune system' was, as they argued, a function of lifestyle. However, what was not understood at the time was that the poor immune system was a result of infection transmitted by a blood-borne virus via sexual and injecting practices, and 'lifestyle' was undefined. It was the specific *social* practices of gay men and of people who inject drugs – engaging in sex with each other and sharing of needles and injection equipment – that placed them at risk of HIV. Although the reference to lifestyles pointed in the right direction, it failed to find any purchase on the cultural and social practices of particular groups, communities or networks. Instead, early biomedical interest into the lifestyles associated with HIV was translated into researching *individual behaviours*.

In this chapter, we chart the early obscuring, by biomedicine, of the notion of *social practice* in the shift in the focus of HIV prevention from groups to individuals and their unsafe or risky *behaviours*. We also describe a more recent turn to 'vulnerable populations' rather than 'risky individuals'. This move to vulnerable populations holds promise: it is an attempt to focus attention on the social and cultural 'drivers' of vulnerability to HIV transmission. As we argue below, the inherent risk of such attempts is that society and culture are understood as structures over which individuals or indeed populations (which epidemiologists understand as comprised of unconnected individuals) have little control. The notion that collective action not only reproduces but *produces* social structures in the form of new social norms and social practices is obscured and overlooked. Approaching the social as a matter of 'structures', where such structures determine behaviours, can make it difficult to understand the agency of people. In particular the agency of 'vulnerable' people becomes virtually impossible to countenance. However, there is an alternative, more productive entry point to HIV prevention.

We argue that HIV prevention requires first an understanding of what groups or collectives, that is, people connected to each other, care about and do. We will show how understanding the shared, and at times, contested, social practices of collectives allows us to see both the ways in which people's lives are shaped by social structures, but also how people's actions contribute to shifts and changes in those same structures as well as to their reproduction. We also argue that understanding collective action requires that HIV prevention efforts replace the notion of 'individual behaviour' with that of 'social practice', and in Chapter 6 we demonstrate that the social practices of groups – that is, communities and networks – and the collective agency of communities are central to both HIV transmission and to the development of effective HIV-prevention strategies.

Risk Groups

With the advent of the HIV test in 1985, rather than having to rely on AIDS cases epidemiologists began their surveillance work to provide the needed information about the patterning of the epidemic(s) – both internationally and within nations. In the years that followed the diagnosis of the young gay man in the United States, HIV was identified in a number of countries, as noted in Chapter 1. In response to the patterning of the epidemic(s) in those early years, epidemiologists set up 'risk categories' in terms of which HIV transmission was understood as an outcome of homosexual sex, injection drug use and so on. These categories conflated practice with group identity[1] and these groups came to be referred to as 'risk groups' (Waldby, 1996). Using 'risk groups' as a way to understand HIV is problematic and creates confusion about HIV transmission; for example, engaging in unprotected anal intercourse with a person living with HIV is what places gay men at risk, not simply 'being gay'. However the use of the concept 'risk groups' also proved unexpectedly beneficial: the outcomes were both 'good' and 'bad'.

On the 'good' side, as we take up and elaborate in Chapter 6, the identification of groups led – at least in some countries – to an engagement with
communities and networks at risk of HIV. Gay communities and networks
of injection drug users and, later, sex workers were supported in a variety of
ways. Governments targeted those communities and networks, either by funding them directly to set up their own HIV-related programmes or by targeting
them with government-run or sanctioned HIV-prevention programmes, thus
enabling them to act to reduce the risk of HIV transmission.

On the 'bad' side, the reliance of HIV epidemiology on the concept of 'risk
group' also led to stigmatisation of these groups, setting up a permeable relationship between HIV epidemiological knowledge and discriminatory practice (Waldby, Kippax & Crawford, 1995). HIV was, and in many countries,
continues to be positioned as the disease of 'the other' – the deviant and the
undeserving. The first such 'risk' group comprised gay men or, as they were
later referred to, men who have sex with men (MSM), quickly followed by
people who inject drugs, referred to as drug users or abusers and, also incor-
rectly, as 'intravenous' drug users.

In the mid to late 1980s, HIV reached Asia, including India, Thailand,
Cambodia, Vietnam and China, and the HIV prevalence data from Asia
also implicated heterosexual transmission, especially among sex workers, as
well as transmission via injection drug use and to a lesser extent homosexual
transmission. Slowly but surely heterosexual transmission was recognised,
although it was initially conceptualised as associated with sex work or sex with
bisexual men or people who inject drugs and, in certain countries with people
from high-prevalence countries, with foreigners. As Altman (2006) points out:
'[T]he reaction in parts of Asia was to brand [HIV] as an American import
and to ban foreigners from places such as bars and nightclubs' (257). Hence,
in the late 1980s and early 1990s, another two groups were added to the list of
'risk groups' so that we now had:

- Gay men
- Injection drug users
- Sex workers
- Foreigners

Notably, although 'sex workers' and 'foreigners' were largely included as some
form of acknowledgement of the fact of heterosexual transmission, the risk
category of 'heterosexuals' is absent. This omission reflects what many did
not want to acknowledge: the possibility of heterosexual transmission of HIV.
Although heterosexual transmission had been documented by the early 1980s
in countries in Africa and elsewhere (Piot, Quinn & Taleman, 1984), there

was considerable argument in public health about it. This debate continued into the middle and late 1980s (see for example, Polk, 1985; Potterat et al., 1987) with some arguing that people who tested HIV-positive were unwilling to say that they injected drugs or were gay. Others down-played the likelihood of transmission in 'normal' heterosexual sex and argued that transmission between heterosexuals occurred because of anal intercourse or, in the case of African epidemics, other 'exotic' practices, such as 'dry sex' (Patton, 2002).

The extent of the difficulty of including 'heterosexuals' in a list of epidemi-ological risk categories is illustrated by the 1990 publication of Fumento's *The Myth of Heterosexual AIDS; How a Tragedy has been Distorted by the Media and Partisan Politics*. In his book, Fumento argued that heterosexuals do get HIV but from unsterile needles, from transfusions, from the clotting factor that people with haemophilia use to control internal bleeding, from their mothers at or before birth, and sometimes from sexual intercourse with persons in these categories or with bisexuals. He argued that HIV was not transmitted from heterosexual to heterosexual (15–16). Of course, some knew that Fumento was wrong, and that what he called a myth was no myth at all. Nonetheless the book had a pow-erful impact, and it was some time before heterosexuals were considered to be at risk. Although the evidence was clearly building, heterosexual transmission of HIV – especially transmission from men to women – was understood to be from gay or bisexual men to women, or to women from men who inject drugs, and HIV transmission from women to men was understood as related to sex work. Alternatively when heterosexuals were seen as a 'risk group', they were 'atypical' heterosexuals and were understood as young (meaning immature) or promiscuous or reckless. This stigmatisation is linked to moralising discourses about AIDS and, in some countries, has had an impact on HIV prevention. In Nigeria, for example, as described recently by Smith (2014), condoms are widely viewed as symbols of sin because the very use of them implies that the user is promiscuous and reckless.

The outcome of this kind of denial and debate was that, in the early 1990s 'women', but not 'heterosexual men', were included as an epidemiological 'risk group' although, interestingly, women were often referred to as an '*at*-risk' group. Other populations were also added later, including young people and prisoners. So these 'risk' or 'at-risk groups' came to include:

- Gay men
- Injection drug users
- Sex workers
- Foreigners
- Women
- Young people

Whether the term 'risk group' or 'at-risk' group is used, the notable absence is the category 'heterosexual men' (Waldby et al., 1993), despite the fact that almost 50 per cent of those living with HIV are men. HIV remains the disease of 'the other'. While it is of utmost importance to acknowledge that gay men, people who inject drugs and sex workers are in special need, the epidemiological and medical focus on 'risk groups' or 'at-risk' groups feeds into and reinforces already existing understandings and stereotypes: normal – deviant, strong – vulnerable, clean – dirty. Heterosexual men seek to cordon off the other and keep themselves safe – creating a 'cordon sanitaire' (1993; Lawless et al., 1996). Stigma and discrimination are reinforced by the epidemiological categories that were developed in order to respond effectively to a virus, a virus that is continuing to spread along societies' fault-lines of race, gender, sexuality and class. As Treichler (1987) noted very early in the epidemic, the very nature of AIDS is constituted through language and, in particular, through the discourses of medicine and science.

Epidemiologists started responding to the criticisms of the confusing and stigmatising nature of 'risk categories' and began replacing the terminology with 'risky behaviours'. Despite this epidemiological turn to 'risk behaviours' (a shift which better fits with epidemiological interest in the movement of disease (Patton, 2002) as opposed to approaching disease as having a fixed location in one group or place), the notion of 'risk groups' or 'at-risk' groups or, politically more correct, 'key populations', is still pervasive in HIV prevention. It has been reinforced by the ways in which HIV surveillance was, and continues to be, carried out: data collected from either mandatory or voluntary testing of particular populations. Although most countries do not pursue mandatory testing, in some countries there was and is mandatory testing of some groups, including returning nationals, resident aliens, aliens entering the country, military personnel, police officers, drug users, sex workers, prisoners, people with haemophilia, pregnant women, children of infected women and patients in hospitals (Mann et al., 1992). The groups undergoing the most frequent compulsory testing were prisoners, followed by those presenting at health care facilities with a sexually transmissible infection, pregnant women, and returning nationals (1992). With regard to HIV surveillance, many countries chose to monitor infections nationally in pregnant women[2] (for example, South Africa) and military recruits (for example, Thailand). These populations are captive and thus provide easy access, and they are also reasonably representative of sexually active populations. Other groups, such as those referred to above, and blood donors provided some sort of triangulation of the surveillance data. Hence, before we turn to the growing use of the concept 'vulnerability' (since 2000) to reframe 'risk', we want to first discuss the relationship between HIV testing and the circulation of notions of 'risk' in HIV prevention.

HIV testing

HIV epidemiology relies on HIV testing and, since 1985, the year the HIV test was developed, people have been urged to test. In 1996, with the development of an effective HIV treatment in the form of ART, HIV testing enabled many with HIV to have access to ART. However, ongoing studies continue to show that HIV testing and stigma are closely associated, affecting people's willingness to test. In a population-based survey of Zambians, although the proportion of people indicating initial willingness to be HIV tested and counselled was 37 per cent, only 3.7 per cent of people came forward for testing, and of these just under half returned for their test results: overall, fewer than 200 of the 4,812 people surveyed (Fylkesnes et al., 1999). Similarly, data from South Africa (cited in Marais, 2005, 33) indicated that in the HSRC 2002 survey less than two-thirds of the respondents identified for the survey agreed to take an HIV test. However, in 2012 just over two-thirds of respondents agreed to do so (Shisana et al., 2014).

These and other studies such as those conducted in Tanzania (Maman et al., 2001; Burke, Rajabu & Kippax, 2004) point to the role of stigma in relation to testing and disclosure. In particular, there are problems for women. Maman et al. (2001) found that the most salient barriers to HIV testing and serostatus disclosure among women they surveyed in Dar es Salaam were fear of their sexual partners' reaction and the undermining of decision-making and communication patterns between partners. Testing itself positions people as 'at risk', and this often means that women are positioned as promiscuous. The work of Grinstead et al. (2001) quantified these fears and problems as negative life events, including breakup of relationships, isolation, exclusion and violence – especially for women. In their study, carried out in Trinidad, Tanzania and Kenya, positive serostatus was associated with the breakup of marriage and being neglected or disowned by the family. Heterosexual serodiscordant couples in which the HIV-positive person was the woman were most likely to report the breakup of a marriage (20% versus 0–7% for other groups) and the breakup of a sexual relationship (45% versus 22–38% for other groups). Physical abuse was also more frequently experienced by HIV-positive women in serodiscordant (13%) and HIV-positive seroconcordant relationships (12%) than in other groups (0–3%). Kalichman & Simbayi (2003) note that stigma is likely to pose considerable barriers to seeking voluntary counselling and testing (VCT) or, more generally, testing, in South Africa – and, given the above, elsewhere in Africa if not further afield.

These negative consequences cannot be explained away as 'teething problems' of the global interest in VCT. A more recent study of pregnant women attending an antenatal clinic in Kenya (Turan et al., 2011) found that, when asked to anticipate a HIV-positive test result, 32 per cent of respondents fore-saw the breakup of their relationship and 45 per cent thought they would lose friends. Furthermore, respondents were more likely to refuse testing if they thought their male partner would react in a discriminatory manner. And a study of MSM in Beijing (Li et al., 2012) found that discriminatory attitudes toward positive people were significant, and that these attitudes were associ-ated with not having had an HIV test oneself.

Clearly, the consequences of HIV testing are complex, and the association with stigma and discrimination needs to be acknowledged and contextually addressed. This need, we argue, is heightened by current efforts to move to TasP. As described in Chapter 4, research between 2008 and 2012 indicated that not only was ART effective, but also that ART acts in a preventive fashion (Vernazza et al., 2008; Cohen et al., 2011). These findings have led to global efforts to roll out and implement TasP – an initiative that requires regular test-ing to identify seroconversion as soon as possible, enabling the early provision of treatment. Clearly HIV testing is central to TasP but how the necessarily high and frequent rates of HIV testing can be achieved lies at the nub of a current dilemma for public health. Although the number of people testing has increased over time, population readiness for testing remains low in many countries, and how this figure can be increased without exacerbating stigma and discrimination remains to be answered. The findings to date indicate that caution is needed, particularly in low- and middle-income countries, because if more stigma and discrimination are created then one of the very reasons for people to test for HIV – increasing access to treatment – will be undermined. Routine HIV testing may be efficient and effective in terms of numbers tested, but in itself it may very well fail to trigger the social change necessary to ensure that people – especially women – are able to test with impunity.

The move to the clinic: 'Risky' individuals

As global efforts to provide access to HIV treatment grew, so too were there expansions in the health service infrastructure and expertise required to test people, counsel those who tested positive, and prescribe and monitor treat-ment. As global funders and institutions interested in HIV prevention watched this developing and growing network of HIV clinics, they began to frame these clinics as bases of expertise from which prevention initiatives could be implemented. In particular, the counselling that people are supposed to receive before and after testing was identified as a site for prevention. Although the value of doubling up on treatment initiatives by adding in prevention efforts might seem obvious when presented in the abstract, it only makes sense if prevention also involves harnessing and addressing communities of people and does not restrict itself only to addressing individuals in the clinic. Yet HIV testing in the clinic is becoming the major, if not the only, site of promoting HIV-prevention strategies, and testing and counselling are being increasingly positioned as the main, if not the only, 'gateway to prevention' along with care, treatment and support. For example, Bekker & Hosek (2015, 3) who, with reference to young people, advise that 'The starting point for all HIV programming commences with counselling and HIV testing'. Prevention has been moved from the everyday world, where people have sex and inject drugs, to the world of the clinic, a shift intensified by the recent push to test and treat. This move has led inexorably to the individualising and privatising of HIV prevention.

Typically, the public health argument for testing as a means of promoting HIV prevention goes as follows: as a responsible, rational, autonomous agent (neo-liberal subject), if you know you are positive you will not engage in unsafe sex, and if you know you are HIV-negative then you will act to remain so. The evidence suggests, however, that matters are not so clear-cut: meta-analyses of available data from a number of studies produce mixed findings with regard to the effectiveness of counselling and testing in reducing HIV-related risk behaviours (Reproductive Health Matters, 2000). The review by Weinhardt et al. (1999), which comprises the findings from a number of studies from the United States (19), Africa (6) and Europe (2), carried out between 1985 and 1997, indicates – notwithstanding an under-reporting of unprotected sex (Allen et al., 2003) – that testing with the associated counselling is not an altogether effective preventive tool. What the evidence indicates is that, although testing and counselling appear to provide an effective means of secondary prevention, that is, decreasing the likelihood of infected individuals infecting others, it does not appear effective in primary prevention: as shown in these studies, uninfected individuals did not reduce their risk behaviour. While the review of the Voluntary HIV-1 Counseling and Testing Efficacy Study Group (2000) indicated a mediocre effect of counselling and testing on risk behaviour, they also found that counselling and testing had greater effectiveness for people who were living with HIV. More recently Denison et al. (2008), in a review of studies conducted in developing countries from 1990 to 2005 also found only moderate effectiveness.

While testing and counselling may work well to *reinforce* HIV-prevention programmes, there is mounting evidence that the inclusion of HIV-prevention education and advice within the context of HIV testing is at best only partially effective. The clinic does not provide the context for effective prevention. HIV counselling as prevention reinforces the notion that HIV transmission is an individual matter, and that people will act to protect themselves and, if they are HIV-positive, to protect others. HIV testing and the move to the clinic has led many countries, particularly the United States, to focus on 'positive prevention' and, hence, on HIV-positive people as responsible for preventing HIV transmission (CDC, 2003). Such a focus carries the risk of undermining the notion of shared responsibility for HIV transmission, dividing communities and increasing stigma and discrimination, particularly in the context of increasing criminalisation of HIV transmission (Kippax & Stephenson, 2012).

Following the recent advances regarding TasP, the focus has shifted to HIV-positive people who have not tested, not taken up ART or have not adhered to their treatment regimens. The potential for stigma and discrimination is obvious. The most recent group singled out for admonition are those people who have not been recently tested or tested at all and, hence, may be at risk of unwittingly transmitting HIV: the 'undiagnosed' (Holt, 2014b). In a very important sense the old, contested, epidemiological ways of framing HIV have recently expanded to designate new notions of 'risky' individuals: HIV-positive people who are not starting treatment early are 'non-adherers', or those HIV-positive people who are unaware of their HIV status, the 'undiagnosed'.

Individualising and privatising prevention

The positioning of the clinic as the *major* site of prevention has led to the individualising and privatising of prevention: it has sidelined efforts to address collectives. Prevention in the clinic is individualistic – at best it entails talking to couples – and, hence, it has little impact on prevailing normative understandings of risk. With regard to sexual transmission, although couples' counselling acknowledges the importance of inserting prevention at the site of the interactions between people, it frames two people's interaction as a matter of rational discussion and, like individual counselling, does not directly target the social norms shaping individuals' and couples' expectations of how sexual relationships are conducted. Similarly, counselling individuals about drug injecting fails to acknowledge, and does not address, the social aspects of injecting with others. Furthermore, in the clinic, HIV-prevention messages are delivered in a 'top down' fashion: people are positioned as patients – as passive recipients of information and advice, not a characteristic of good, effective education. Such positioning is disempowering. Little if any attention is given to the ways in which the testing and counselling messages are interpreted and understood by those who receive them. Because, in the clinic, those tested and counselled are positioned as 'patients', prevention also risks pathologising them. Those who are HIV-positive are positioned as primarily responsible for infection, and such positioning reinforces notions of blame and shame and, more generally, stigma and discrimination.

Even more importantly, and perhaps most importantly, positioning testing as a major prevention tool gives governments the excuse to draw back from the social practices involved in HIV transmission, offers the excuse not to have to deal with and face the complexities of talking about sex and drugs, the excuse not to train teachers and those in contact with young people to raise issues in connection with HIV transmission. It excises the public and collective voice (Kippax, 2006). It privatises sexual matters and the use of illegal drugs and thereby enables governments to leave, untroubled, the hegemonic power structures – gender, sexuality, race and class – that are the very structures that aid in the transmission of HIV and that need addressing and reworking as part of HIV prevention.

In general, this move to the clinic positions the 'risky' or 'at-risk' individual as the potential agent of change and sidelines and undermines the collective, the community or network, as the site of change. 'Risk' groups or 'key' populations are understood as comprised of unconnected individuals: neo-liberal subjects, who, it is assumed will act rationally in their own best interest. Little if any attention is paid to the social relations between people who have sex together or inject drugs and share needles and injection equipment, and there is no understanding that social norms enable and regulate the social practices in which people engage. It is the social norms and social practices that are in need of change. As discussed in Chapter 4, whether prevention programmes or interventions advocate the use of condoms, clean needles and syringes, microbicides or pre- and post-exposure prophylaxis or testing and treating, they all require changes in practice. Furthermore, with the exception of male circumcision, they all require changes that have to be sustained over time. Condoms have to be used or microbicide gels applied (or both) every time one has sex, and clean needles and syringes used every time one injects drugs. The latest in technological innovation, testing and treating all with HIV infection ('test and treat' or TasP), also requires changes in practice: annual or more frequent HIV testing for those who test HIV-negative and, for those who test HIV-positive and accept early treatment, a life-long regimen of drugs, many of which have short- and long-term side effects. Such changes in social practice are a function of widespread social change which, in turn, is produced by collective action – not by changes in each and every individual's behaviour. Social change is unlikely to be the outcome of interventions targeted at individuals or couples, particularly if the interventions are confined to the clinic.

Vulnerable Populations

While the notion of 'risk' was the main focus of early prevention efforts, in the 1990s some Global HIV and AIDS researchers and policy advisors began to acknowledge and design programmes to address the inadequacies of HIV-prevention efforts targeting the risky behaviours of individuals – typically positioned as rational, autonomous agents (Mann, Tarantola & Netter, 1992). The 2000 World AIDS Report marked a watershed moment in having UNAIDS highlight and seek to address the limitations of framing HIV transmission as a matter of 'risk':

> Individuals do not live and make decisions in a vacuum. After years of focusing on personal choices about lifestyles, by the early 1990s AIDS prevention programmes were giving renewed attention to the social and economic context of people's daily lives. [...] Recognition of the factors that fuel the HIV epidemic prompted the development of new programmes for reducing vulnerability – in the civil, political, economic, social and cultural arenas – that would work in synergy with the more traditional prevention approaches aimed at diminishing risk-taking behavior. (UNAIDS, 2000, 37)

This report signalled the adoption of 'vulnerability' by UNAIDS and the World Health Organization (WHO); the traditional object of HIV intervention, individual risk behaviour, was supplemented with a new object, 'vulnerability' (Ayres, Paiva & Franca, 2011).

The emphasis on vulnerability in the 2000 World AIDS Report represented an attempt to support HIV-prevention efforts that addressed the *social* 'factors', 'contexts', 'structures' or (more commonly discussed now as) 'drivers' shaping HIV transmission patterns and responses to it. This move was clearly informed by the work of Farmer. An anthropologist and physician, Farmer (1992; Farmer, Connors & Simmons, 1996) had earlier turned public health's attention to the structures, the fault lines, implicated in the transmission of HIV. With reference to Haiti, he describes the close links between 'unimaginable poverty' (which he accounts for in terms of the gross social and economic inequalities produced by neo-liberal economies, especially those of France and the United States), and HIV prevalence and AIDS deaths. Among others, Farmer argued that prevention efforts aiming to reduce 'vulnerability' to HIV transmission needed to target the structures shaping that vulnerability. The notion of 'vulnerability' and the associated notion of 'structural violence' (Farmer, 2004) began to be taken up in HIV-related public health research. Since 2000, the problem of vulnerability, understood as produced by social and economic structural forces, has increasingly shaped efforts to understand and address HIV transmission in concert with efforts addressing individual risk-taking behaviours.

It should be noted that there is a long history of public health interest in things other than individual behaviours and lifestyles. In the nineteenth and early twentieth centuries, public health largely focused on contexts – typically environmental or physical contexts rather than social or cultural ones. Understanding contexts in this way enabled public health to intervene by, for example, providing clean water and sanitation or by pushing for policy or legislation to improve housing and living conditions (Cosgrave, Fairchild & Rosner, 2013). In contemporary public health, such efforts to improve health by directly tackling environmental factors or by developing policies to address the 'structural factors' shaping living conditions are ongoing. As Sommer & Parker point out (2013, 2), public health most often 'conceptualize[s] structural and environmental factors as aspects of health policy and institutional programmes and practices that influence the context in which health behaviours take place'. Importantly, this meant then (and in some quarters continues to mean) that it is possible to have a public health discussion of the structures affecting daily living conditions without discussing the *social* structures that social scientists research. As we argue below, public health researchers often underplay the role of social structures. When they do attend to structures, the social becomes a context in which the behaviours of individuals are determined or driven. The term 'vulnerability' that emerged from social epidemiology becomes the property of individuals or populations composed of unconnected individuals who are made vulnerable because of outside forces, or 'drivers'.

Social drivers

Notwithstanding the shifting meanings of 'structure' (as contexts or factors that determine or drive or influence or shape behaviours), the move to address *social* structures is important. In 2011 and in 2012 two special issues were devoted to the role of social structures, or drivers, in HIV transmission. In 2012 a special issue of the *Journal of the International AIDS Society* highlighted the importance of sustaining efforts to address social structures in responding to HIV (Seeley et al., 2012). The authors of this special issue take Auerbach et al.'s definition of social drivers as its starting point: 'core social processes and arrangements – reflective of social and cultural norms, values, networks, structures and institutions, that operate in concert with individuals' behaviours and practices to influence HIV epidemics in particular settings' (2011, S294–295). Most of the papers in the 2012 supplement are devoted to empirical research and many also refer to earlier empirical work. The studies interrogate the relationships between social structures and HIV transmission and demonstrate connections between inequities in gender and power relations and socio-economic status, on the one hand, and vulnerability to HIV, on the other (Mbonye et al., 2012; Macpherson et al., 2012; Gibbs et al., 2012; Hargreaves et al., 2012). While most of these same studies also point to (and many suggest) possible structural interventions to reduce vulnerability to HIV, one paper (Hargreaves et al., 2012) exemplifies the mixed success of efforts to address vulnerability with reference to supporting girls' greater participation in education, gender empowerment and micro-finance and financial literary interventions (echoing Dworkin and Blankenship's 2009 review of micro-finance interventions among women and girls). In the same special issue, Gibbs et al. (2012) point to the lessons learned from their review of structural interventions, and Parkhurst (2012) offers a framework to overcome problems in structural HIV-prevention approaches, which we take up below and in Chapter 6.

The other special issue was published a year earlier, in 2011, in the journal *Global Public Health*, with a focus on vulnerability. The content was authored by the Social Drivers Group, one of nine multi-disciplinary working groups set up by UNAIDS in 2007 to address concerns with the state of HIV prevention. The papers address the structural factors or social 'drivers' that produce or 'drive' vulnerability. As described in the introductory paper of this special supplement (Ogden et al., 2011), the social-drivers approach can be distinguished from other prevention approaches by its focus on reducing vulnerability rather than individual risk. They define 'vulnerability' as

> a sociological concept that refers to the extent to which the risk of transmission is affected by factors in the broader social and/or physical environment, which may be *beyond the control of any or all individuals* involved. Specifically, the concept has been used to explain why individuals fail to respond with apparent rationality (that is in ways that seem to protect their own best interests) to HIV prevention programming focused on individual risk reduction. (Ogden et al., 2011, S286, emphasis added)

It is notable here that social structures are positioned as things that may be *beyond* the grasp of individuals. We highlight this because, although the work on social drivers explicitly sets out to understand how communities and groups can actively respond to HIV as it affects them and so take some control, it is common for public health to separate social determinants, or structures, from individual control, or agency. Consider also the definition of vulnerability as given in the 2011 UNAIDS Terminology Guidelines:

> Vulnerability refers to unequal opportunities, social exclusion, unemployment, or precarious employment, and other social, cultural, political, and economic factors that make a person more susceptible to HIV infection and to developing AIDS. The factors underlying vulnerability may reduce the ability of individuals and communities to avoid HIV risk and may be *outside the control of individuals*. (UNAIDS, 2011, 30, emphasis added)

These definitions usefully underscore that inequalities related to gender, race, sexuality, and socio-economic differences play a central role, not only in the manner in which HIV is transmitted, but also in the ways in which populations are able to respond to HIV. They acknowledge the importance of advocacy for addressing inequalities through national government actions and local initiatives, including community-based organising and action. They also raise an important question: How can people tackle something 'beyond individual control'? However, without an entry point for understanding and thinking about what happens *between* 'social structures' and 'individual control', the separation or opposition evoked here can hinder rather than assist the design of HIV-prevention programmes that target social norms and social practice. Hence, the challenge for social scientists, public health and biomedical researchers alike, is to find ways to acknowledge, think about and work on social structures, factors or drivers without closing down the possibility of thinking about how groups of people are involved in *changing* social norms and social practices.

Returning to the Social Drivers Working Group's supplement: we can see something of their concern with opening up this middle ground when Ogden and colleagues frame structural approaches to HIV prevention as creating the conditions in which people can make healthy choices: '[T]hey reduce vulnerability and foster *resilience* at the individual level; at the collective level they support the development of *AIDS-competent communities*' (Ogden et al., 2011, S286).

In introducing the notion of 'resilience', the Social Drivers Working Group attempts to take account of people's collective action, action instanced by the early effective responses to HIV in countries such as Australia and Uganda. Resilience, they argue, results from the 'dynamic interplay between individual agency and AIDS-competent communities' (Ogden et al., 2011, S287) and 'is in place when *individuals* are able to manage the risks that are present in their environment' (2011, S287, emphasis added). Resilience appears to be described as an individual capacity first and foremost, albeit one that is shaped by structures.

> The Social Drivers Working Group understands individuals as active agents in the creation of their own well-being, but sees capacity as being influenced by critical elements in the social structure, such as norms and values, economic, political and (other) social institutions and networks. Such concrete attributes as knowledge and skills, access to information and resources are also critical dimensions of agency. (Ogden et al., 2011, S287)

We see here the familiar separation of the two poles of 'individual' and 'social structure'. Such a separation is so familiar that it is taken for granted by many.

However, we want to emphasise again that the difficulty with such 'common-sense' is that the ways in which *groups* of people are actively involved in making and re-making norms, values, economic, political and (other) social institutions and networks are not foregrounded. The result of this absence is that the very object of interest – that is, the processes that are in play to produce resilience – are not opened up for interrogation. How AIDS-competent communities become competent, and how such communities are produced by or produce 'resilient' individuals is missing. Furthermore, the interpersonal and social factors invoked in this account appear to be independent of, and beyond the control of, individuals: there is little sense that, collectively, individuals or persons can and do act on occasion to produce social structures.

The social drivers approach of thinking HIV prevention as a matter of addressing 'vulnerability' in place of 'risk', while crucial, does not take us far enough in the effort to conceive of and work with collective agency. Although 'resilience' might invoke a strengths-based, as opposed to a deficit-based, mode of responding (Baum, 2008), there is no account of the ways in which resilience is produced in AIDS-competent communities or, at best, such accounts are incomplete.

There is an awareness of these problems in both special supplements and the papers, which acknowledge that addressing HIV vulnerability is a long-term project: there is no quick fix. They also foreground the complexity of the social and political issues likely to be involved and the difficulties of designing effective prevention that targets the social drivers of HIV: the complexity and associated challenges arising from the fact that 'social forces do not operate in the same way in every setting' (Ogden et al., 2011, S289). Understanding this specificity, they argue, means that sociological analysis of the local and particular are necessary – and both this analysis and the design of any initiative demands 'genuinely engaging with affected communities' (S290). Acknowledging this specificity also puts paid to any notion of a linear causal relationship between prevention interventions and outcomes: the effect of interventions is a contingent matter. Gibbs et al. (2012), in raising issues in relation to attending to the *particular* social factors, also warn against too-narrow a conceptualisation of social factors and contend that it is essential to work closely with organisations that have local, contextual or insider knowledge. They also argue that current approaches to HIV vulnerability may not be 'upstream' enough and may fail to challenge the wider social, political and economic constraints under which many people live. Pointing to a distinction between 'proximal' and 'distal' social structures, Gibbs et al. (2012) suggest that HIV prevention needs to address both.

Although these researchers and authors point to the importance of community, and the Social Drivers Working Group discuss AIDS-competent communities, there is a real sense in much of this work that vulnerability and resilience are the properties of individuals. The interplay between communities (competent or not) and individuals (resilient or not) is not fully discussed. Furthermore, we suggest that the concept of 'resilience' as it is so pervasively used in public health today, might usefully invoke a strengths-based mode of connecting to communities, while simultaneously delimiting what those strengths, or collective agency, might entail. Resilience invokes communities as active in the face of the threat of HIV or other public health challenges, and as responsible for effecting solutions. Yet, any collective action is pre-framed as a response to the problem as it has already been identified by public health or by those involved in funding, designing and implementing responses (Neocleous, 2013). Once framed this way, actions such as those taken by HIV-positive men in the 1980s – undermining the randomised controlled trials of drug efficacy in which they were trial participants by testing the drugs to identify whether they were in the experimental or placebo arms and by sharing drugs within non-trial participants who could not access the drugs any other way – may not count as 'resilience'. The collective action of communities that fail to be persuaded to take part in mass testing because they are reasonably informed that the process may increase discrimination likewise may not count as 'resilience'. The concept of resilience does not interrupt hasty interpretations of people's unexpected or undesired actions (from the perspective of HIV-prevention practitioners or researchers) to be the result of 'misunderstanding' or 'lack of agency'. Thus, like vulnerability, resilience curtails public health engagement with people's collective agency – agency that manifests as questioning the limits of HIV prevention as it has been imagined and implemented to date.

While the Social Drivers Working Group does foreground the importance of agency, their conceptualisation of agency still needs elaboration beyond notions of individual agency. In general, the contemporary turn to 'vulnerability' on the part of global HIV prevention problematically positions the individual members of vulnerable populations as passive victims and incapable of action. Yet, the focus on the vulnerable, or the oppressed, risks turning attention away from the forces of oppression, and instead making the 'targeted' members of such vulnerable populations responsible.

The absence of collective agency

These moves beyond 'risk categories' and the 'individual' so as to include social relations and structures are vitally important. There has been – at least in some quarters – a re-engagement with the social worlds of people affected by, and at risk of, HIV infection. However, as suggested above, extending the focus of HIV prevention beyond individuals (and beyond 'risk behaviour') amplifies some important challenges – in particular the challenge of under-standing, recognising and working with the ways groups of people can exercise agency over their lives, developing more effective responses to the epidemic as it presents itself to them. Notwithstanding Farmer's (2004) warning that one should not romanticise resistance to oppression, the notion of 'vulnerability' currently in use in most biomedical and some social-science narratives of HIV positions people and communities as passive and unable to act (and so in need of some external force to 'enable' them). While it is true that individuals are unlikely to be able to avoid HIV risk as an individual alone, together they can and indeed have done so.

We must move beyond a reductionist understanding of structural vio-lence as something that comes from an external source and works along lin-ear, deterministic pathways forcing people to respond. Certainly, at the local level, 'everyday life is shaped by the historical processes and contemporary politics of global political economy' but, as Bourgois & Scheper-Hughes (2004, 318) suggest, the continuum of constraints and violence that people encounter are also shaped by local cultures in which people actively participate to make, re-make and re-work social norms and practices. Although it may well be the case in countries such as Haiti that structural violence is such that collective agency is extremely difficult, if not impossible, it can and does occur as demonstrated in Uganda and Australia (Chapters 2 and 3). Understand-ing such events demands that the notion of agency needs to be broadened to include *collective agency*, which arises out of social relations between people and the social practices of collectives or communities (Altman, 1994). Recognising and understanding collective agency also demands that our engagement with what people are experiencing and doing at the local level be attuned to mean-ings and practices that may not be expected. That is, we may encounter col-lective agency in forms that easily align with a pre-conceived notion of what 'resilient' community action might look like (for example, the broad uptake of condoms), but collective agency might also be expressed in the form of experi-mental, unproven ways (to public health's eyes) of navigating the challenges of the epidemic, such as Australia's gay communities' early pro-sex responses with the adoption of condom use at a time *before* the effectiveness of condoms had been recognised by public health, and their resistance to pleas by public health to reduce the number of their sexual partners.

The embracing of vulnerability has often had the unintended conse-quence of making agency disappear, almost by definition, because vulner-ability assumes that people cannot act until the social is changed and, more importantly, rendering agency ungraspable without an understanding that it is often the so-called vulnerable who initiate the needed change. Thus, in public health, this approach is of limited use in promoting what it often sets out to do (that is, grass-roots HIV-prevention efforts), because such efforts begin with social *relations*. Approaching the social in the form of problematic social structures or barriers invites vertical, or top-down, attempts to deal with or tackle the social on behalf of the vulnerable. Instead of stimulating resistance in the face of structural violence, HIV-prevention premised vulnerability may become immobilising because of the seemingly insurmountable task of transforming macro-level social structures that lie beyond the reach of even the largest public health programmes (Farmer, 2004; Farmer, Connors & Simmons, 1996; Parker, 1996, 2002). Indeed, there is a real risk that the focus on vulnerability/resilience enables public health and biomedicine to avoid community and, in so doing, social structures are not understood as something that people collectively can and do transform. As Krieger (2008) argues, it is not the case that proximal factors (those close to the individual) 'cause' or determine HIV transmission, nor is it the case that upstream distal factors do so. Rather, as she says: 'The distal and the proximal are conjoined' (224). They may curtail action, but possibilities exist for people to exercise power over both.

The disjuncture between people and society

Although the Social Drivers Working Group does foreground the central importance of community (as in their notion of AIDS-competent communities), by conceiving of HIV prevention as targeting HIV vulnerability they do not counter ways of thinking about 'vulnerability' that invoke a false dualism between people and their societies. Without a strong concept of collective agency, we cannot fully grasp how people by their actions, reproduce and produce societies or how AIDS-competent communities develop.

In the absence of any investigation of the social relations that connect people to each other, attributes of a population are mistakenly conflated with and addressed as attributes of individuals within that population (Williams, 2003). Although the move to the notion of vulnerability originates as a move to extend beyond the idea of individual behaviour, the notion of an individual is still problematically prioritised over and above recognition or understanding of what connects people to each other, and what forms the stuff of their social and cultural lives. The benefits of addressing vulnerability are described in a way that augments the same subject: the rational, individual agent of liberal and neoliberal societies is upheld as the ideal mode of being. Thus, criticisms of assumptions about the limits of the autonomous subject – who is invoked when behaviour is the main object of research or intervention – are reinterpreted (and misinterpreted) to mean if only the social and political conditions were right we would all be in a position to have our behaviour targeted by well-designed health interventions, and we would all act rationally and take up the technologies promoted (Auerbach, Parkhurst & Caceres, 2011).

However, there is real promise here and, as we discuss in the following chapter, concepts such as 'social capital' – as used by Thomas-Slayter & Fisher (2011), also members of the Social Drivers Working Group – offer a way forward. In Chapter 6 we discuss how 'being vulnerable' does not necessarily mean that responding to HIV is outside the control of persons, at least as understood as connected to one another in communities. Indeed, being vulnerable has *triggered* many persons, as members of communities and networks, to act in such a way as to change and transform the social worlds they inhabit.

Conclusions

Although HIV presents a difficult target, we do know what works – however imperfectly. The evidence discussed in this book indicates that changes in practices associated with sex and injection drugs are aided and abetted by community activism, political will and structural change – such as the introduction of anti-discrimination laws. Widespread and sustained social change is highly unlikely to occur without engaging the social relations between people and the social worlds they inhabit.

Individuals do change their actions but, typically, via changes in the collective, the community. Indeed, if it were otherwise, HIV prevention would be extremely difficult, in that each and every individual would have to be counselled and advised. The importance of the social milieu in changing people's behaviour cannot be underestimated, as demonstrated, for example, in brainwashing. As researchers studying the effects of imprisonment in isolation have shown, changing beliefs, values and practices that people deem important to them only seems to occur after very long periods in isolation from their fellow prisoners (Segal, 1954; Lifton, 1954; Schein, 1958; Shallice, 1972). Sustained change in an individual's beliefs and behaviours is extremely difficult if the social values and norms of that individual's community and networks, values that connect him or her to others, are different from those that are the object of change.

Until the mid-1990s, many of the changes that made sex and injecting safe, or safer, were a product of the actions of communities and groups supported by governments. The move to the clinic, which was associated with the landmark discovery of effective treatment in 1996, has unwittingly undermined what communities did best – HIV prevention. Clinics, by their very nature, do not engage with communities but speak to individuals or, at best, couples. Although it is important for physicians, nurses and counsellors to reinforce HIV-prevention messages, it is a mistake to assume that HIV prevention delivered via the clinic is the answer to preventing HIV transmission. A public voice is needed – not only a private one.

The return in the early 2000s to the social worlds in which people have sex and inject drugs was much needed. However, this return has been and continues to be a fraught one, in part because the connections between people have been overlooked, and the ways in which people (via those connections) both produce as well as reproduce their social worlds have been forgotten. The focus on structures, or drivers – such as socio-economic status, livelihood insecurity, gender inequality and access to education – is of vital importance. However, changes in these structures not only take time, but they also rely on the collective actions of people. There is an important sense in which such a focus on structures and drivers can disempower people unless it is done in tandem with a robust understanding of what empowers people – collective action.

This is not only an abstract, theoretical concern. In many countries, HIV prevention has become the business of large, international non-governmental organisations (INGOs), such as UNAIDS and WHO and governments and large national entities working internationally, such as the US President's Emergency Plan for AIDS Relief (PEPFAR). Through their focus on 'vulner-ability', the job of the INGOs has become to point out the 'social barriers' that they believe make it impossible for rational individual agents to act in the appropriate manner to protect themselves. The risk here is that the communities affected by HIV are sidelined and forgotten.

HIV prevention is increasingly understood as something comprised of information imparted from doctor or counsellor to individual 'patient', and as something that INGOs and governments do to enable individuals to act on the advice of their doctor or counsellor. The people who inhabit the social and cultural worlds in which HIV is transmitted and prevented are forgotten. More importantly, the role people play as members of collectives in trans-forming their social practices and the social norms that enable and regulate such practices in producing social change is made invisible. We discuss how to put people, not 'individuals', back into HIV prevention in Chapter 6.

Chapter 6

SOCIAL PRACTICES OF COMMUNITIES

This chapter offers a way beyond the apparent impasse between (individualistic) HIV-prevention efforts focused on individual risk behaviours and attempts to target the social drivers of HIV transmission, which fail to adequately account for collective agency. We have argued that there is much to be elucidated between the two poles of 'individual' and 'social structure' and, furthermore, unless we develop our understanding and ways of working with this middle ground of social practices we cannot fully grasp how social change occurs in ways that matter for HIV prevention. Hence, here we turn to this middle ground and examine *how* social practices can transform social structures, including norms – in more or less useful ways for HIV prevention – and consider when and how social practice might fail to trigger much change at all.

Our point of departure is that persons or people typically act as members of collectives. They are essentially social beings (Harré, 1979). People take up the social practices that make sense to others (that is, not only to themselves) in their group or community: for example, as condom use does in many gay communities. Such practices are produced in the social relations among people: it is in these relations that people's actions acquire meaning and norms are appropriated and sustained. As Harré (1979, 125) argues, people's actions are directed to practical social ends, to maintaining the material and social world, and they are also directed to expressive presentations to show what sort of person they are. For instance, for many in gay communities in the 1980s and early 1990s, condoms were used to enable 'safe sex', and they were also used to demonstrate one's concern for others and one's belonging to gay community (Weeks, 1998). If condom use becomes the norm within a particular group, it may be difficult to engage in unprotected sex.

Using condoms, reducing the number of one's sexual partners, using sterile needles and syringes and taking prophylactic drugs are all social practices: these practices, which comprise a sequence of actions that constitute 'sexual engagement' or 'injection drug use', are understood with reference to social norms, rules and conventions, that is, social structures. And these social structures enable people to act, as well as constrain the actions of people. As with the instructions for a recipe or the rules of a soccer game, social norms regulate 'how' to act, what is appropriate and what is not and enable particular types of outcomes. We can be reasonably assured about what those outcomes might entail, according to Harré (1979), depending on whether we are engaging in a ritual social practice, a routine social practice or a game. The endpoint of a ritual can be anticipated – for example, if two people utter the words of their marriage vows (in the appropriate context) the result is that they will be married. Similarly, routine practices, such as queuing at an automatic bank teller, inserting a bank card and the appropriate PIN numbers and requesting cash out of one's account ordinarily has a fairly predictable outcome (if the cash is there). A game is somewhat different: the rules of a soccer match dictate how people will play (or be sanctioned if the rules are not followed), but neither the sequence of events nor final score can be predicted in advance. Thinking of the social practices entailed in injection drug use and sex, there are ritualised, routinised and playful practices. Consider the social practices emerging via gay men's use of online hook up devices (discussed in Chapter 3). Race's (2014b, 2015) account of the emerging practices of 'party and play' details how online discussions about HIV status, viral load and preferences for specific sexual acts (including condom use or not) are becoming routine elements of negotiating hook ups prior to meeting. The relative openness of sexual 'play' is then enabled by a shared understanding of what social practices might be entailed in the hook up, shaping how people interact with each other.

Rules or norms are reproduced in people's practices, but they can also be modified via people's social interactions: they are not fixed – as demonstrated in the changes to Ugandans' and Australian gay men's sexual practices, discussed in Chapters 2 and 3. Communities can and do transform the social worlds in which they live; they can and do change their social practices, and new structures, institutions and norms are produced. Persons can exercise agency, that is, their actions are not wholly determined by outside forces, and they can and do resist the social norms that regulate their practices. However it is collective agency, produced via social capital and through social interactions and talk, which brings about social change and the modification of social practices. As we demonstrate in this chapter, the evidence suggests that HIV prevention is effective when it is grounded in communities – such as gay communities, friendship groups or social networks. It is by working with collective agency that social practices of communities were and continue to be transformed: condoms were adopted, sterile needles and syringes used, sexual partner numbers reduced and prophylactic drugs used. People, via their actions, produce as well as reproduce their social worlds.

There are a number of concepts that are central to any understanding of how the social worlds of people are reproduced and changed. First, rather than focus on 'risk behaviours' of irrational or ill-informed individuals, understanding social change requires a focus on the specific social practices and modes of 'collective agency' that give rise to new or modified practices. Second, in place of directly examining 'vulnerable populations' and the macro-social structures that render these populations vulnerable, researching social change necessitates recognising communities and the kinds of social capital that exist and enable the transformation of people's social worlds. Related to this point, we need to specify how we understand social structures such that is possible to take a realistic (rather than idealistic) approach to how they change. Social structures are often approached as 'macro' (as opposed to 'micro' or 'meso'). Macro-level structures such as gender norms or socio-economic differentiation lead to structural inequalities across an entire society and have been invoked by large bureaucratic organisations (such as the Joint United Nations Programme on HIV/AIDS (UNAIDS) as determinants of HIV transmission and thus in need of change. Such macro social structures can appear to be literally beyond the reach of ordinary people. Change seems impossible. However, these so-called macro structures can be, and are, resisted and changed by entities and actors operating at the meso level. As noted by Krieger (2008) and referred to in Chapter 5, the proximal (micro) and the distal (macro) are conjoined, although Krieger warns against using the term 'levels', at the meso level. The middle ground provides the appropriate focus for effective HIV prevention.

Social norms related to gender and socio-economic status operate at the meso level and are reproduced and modified by people as they *interact with each other* as members of communities (for example, of ethnically based identity groups), or political parties or factions, or a peak body representing non-governmental organisations (NGOs) involved in HIV prevention in a country or state. The Treatment Action Campaign (TAC) in South Africa provides an example of how norms with regard to treatment access were changed by community-level activism, and other examples are discussed in this chapter. Thus, as we show below, it is by identifying how social structures are produced and reproduced at the meso level that it is possible to recognise how social structures do change, and to work in ways that help produce that change where it is needed. In this chapter these concepts – of social practice, collective agency and community – are elaborated to give a detailed account of the ways in which effective HIV prevention works.

Social Practice

As some researchers have pointed out – some as early as 1991 – the use of the term 'risk behaviour' has limited value because it fails to identify the factors that produce the 'behaviour' (Zwi & Cabral, 1991). The problem lies as much, if not more so, with the concept of 'behaviour' as with the concept of 'risk'. Over the past twenty years, as social epidemiology has provided more and more information, especially HIV prevalence and behavioural surveillance data, attention has slowly moved to identify particular patterns of risk behaviours in particular settings (regions or countries) and times (Buve et al., 2002; Chen et al., 2007; Grassly et al., 2003; Ruxrungtham et al., 2004; Wellings et al., 2006). Recognising such patterns can usefully lead to questions about the meaning of particular acts or actions in one time in place, questions that point us towards discussing social practices. Social research and epidemiological studies have highlighted a number of particular forms of sexual practice as risk behaviours, including multi-partner sex and concurrent partnering; paid or transactional sex; homosexual or gay sexual partnering; and in some countries and regions, marital sex or sex between regular partners. Similarly, with regard to injecting drugs, what places people who inject drugs at risk is the sharing of needles and syringes. Although these acts can be abstracted and patterns discerned, these abstractions may not elucidate what people understand themselves to be doing, because people always act with reference to meaning, which typically is specific to the particular social context. Hence, what places communities and populations at risk are practices, not behaviours (Kippax & Stephenson, 2005; Kippax, 2008). And because HIV-prevention efforts need to make sense to people and engage with what they are doing, effective HIV prevention demands that we understand and work with practices. Here we should say that interrogating social practices involves examining the ways in which social, cultural and, as Race (2015) points out, technological factors give rise to and produce particular practices. This understanding enables the identification of how practices are being or might be changed. Sexual or drug injection behaviours are patterned and organised with reference to normative understandings and discourses. Their meanings are formed in the relations between people with reference to the interpersonal contexts and networks in which they are enacted and in response to prevailing socio-cultural, economic and political structures. To illustrate using the example of sexual behaviour, the most powerful influences on human sexuality are social norms – comprised of morals, taboos, laws, beliefs as well as material entities such as contraception – that regulate, enable and govern its expression. Although sexual behaviours may be similar across time and place, sexual practice differs. There are only a small number of different sexual behaviours in which two or more people can engage: sexual intercourse (both vaginal and anal), oral-genital sex (fellatio and cunnilingus) and oral-anal sex; a number of more esoteric behaviours, such as sadomasochism, as well as a range of behaviours that involve touching, mutual masturbatory behaviours.

Sexual practice, on the other hand, is far more fluid: it has a number of forms. Sexual practice is fundamentally social and cultural, being produced within a particular historical time and place and embedded in specific locations and social formations. Sexual practice is different in Australia than in France or Botswana; it was different in medieval times and the 1970s than now. It differs depending upon whether it is enacted within a stable relationship or a casual encounter and whether it is imposed, as in rape, or mutually agreed upon. It is different for men and for women and for heterosexuals and for homosexuals. Sexual practice differs in terms of its location with respect to the prevailing discourses or common understandings that relate to sexuality, love, intimacy, pleasure, reproduction and so on and to the positions that people take up with respect to these discourses. Particular sexual spaces and contexts give rise to particular types of sexual encounters with their own protocols and expectations of participants (Race, 2015).

The distinction between 'practice' and 'behaviour' is crucial. People do not 'do' behaviours, such as penis-in-vaginal sex. They engage in sexual practices: they make love, they 'hook up', they 'party and play', they 'lose their virginity', they work/pay for sex, and so forth. Marital sex, for example, is governed and regulated by social norms: in many cultures, the sexual partners in a marital relationship are expected to be faithful to one another, and sex outside the marital relationship is considered adulterous and in some cultures punishable by death. It is engaged in within long-lasting forms of cohabitation, typically between a man and a woman, and typically it is the site of reproduction.

Some of these sexual practices are safer than others with respect to HIV transmission, but it is vital to make realistic rather than moralistic appraisals of safety. For example, if absolutely monogamous, marital sex is safe with regard to HIV transmission – at least, if both partners are HIV-negative. Within marital relationships governed by norms of fidelity, condom use is unlikely – particularly if sex within marriage is shaped by social norms that emphasise reproduction. This means that if the two conditions – initial HIV-negative seroconcordance and monogamy – are not met then, as we saw in Chapter 2 in Uganda in the early 2000s, marital relationships can constitute a significant site for HIV transmission. Similarly, many regard 'party and play' (that is, casual sexual encounters between gay men organised via mobile phone apps) as unsafe. However, as Race (2015) points out and we elaborate below, online interactions that lead to sexual engagement can often facilitate disclosure of HIV serostatus and, if HIV-positive, level of viral load. Such information can and does inform participants' judgments of HIV-transmission risk. There are multiple HIV-prevention strategies in play in attempts to arrange safe sex. Such practices are clearly made and remade by social norms and material technologies.

The malleability of social practice

How social practices are made and remade is not a matter for 'rational individual agents' who make decisions to act. Nor is it a deterministic process driven by social factors completely outside people's control. Rather, the reproduction and transformation of social practices hinges on collective agency. The 'party and play' scenario underscores the 'agency' of those involved: a collective agency produced through the interactions and practices of gay social bonds and community life, whether that community be online or 'real'.

As noted in Chapter 3, condom use among gay men is an example of changing sexual practices. Condom use as an HIV-prevention strategy was initiated and developed by gay men in the United States and was subsequently appropriated by gay communities around the world via experimentation, discussion and talk, and the input of community agencies and – in some places – governments, which supplied condoms and endorsed their use. In the early 1980s, the practice of condom use among gay men in high-income countries, such as Australia, was enabled by the vibrancy of gay culture: gay men had already come together in the 1960s and 1970s and formed close-knit communities to advocate for gay rights (Smith, 2005). The existence of these community ties enabled early effective responses to the threat of HIV. That is, these gay communities can be seen as AIDS-competent communities, or as becoming AIDS-competent (Campbell, 2010): prior to the threat of HIV they had acquired advocacy and lobbying skills during their political struggle and, in the face of HIV, there was a desire for the community to remain strong and not succumb to the ravages of AIDS. Peer leaders sought out information by reading medical literature on HIV; they consulted specialist HIV medical practitioners, many of whom were gay men; and they remained abreast of HIV research. This information was then circulated in communities by publishing accessible summaries in the gay press and by publicly discussing new information as it became available. Sexual practices were changed and became safer.

There are many accounts of the emergence of other forms of sexual practices in attempts to respond to HIV. In many countries, including Uganda, people reduced the number of their sexual partners. As HIV testing became common in many countries people began to serosort, restricting their sexual engagements to those who had the same serostatus as themselves. Indeed, as mentioned, in Malaysia in 2009 HIV testing became mandatory for couples before marriage (Burns, 2009). While there are risks involved in serosorting – for example, one may not know one's own or one's partner's current serostatus – a relatively safe form of serosorting emerged in Australia (as discussed in Chapter 3) in the mid-1980s: the practice of 'negotiated safety'.

Negotiated safety arose out of the interactions between gay men in Australia, and its practice was based on gay men's knowledge of the biomedical literature and on their knowledge of gay life: a social and cultural capital (Bourdieu, 1986). It is a deliberate strategy on the part of some gay men to dispense with condoms within their regular committed relationships without necessarily giving up sex or anal intercourse outside the relationship. It is not a strategy imposed from the outside but one grounded in the discussion and talk between men and was strengthened and reinforced by an Australian HIV/ AIDS community organisation (ACON) with funding from the government health department. The safe adoption of such a practice involves communication, talk, familiarity and ease with one's sexual partner – and trust, but not necessarily fidelity. Armed with this information and the funding, ACON developed a campaign called *Talk Test Test Trust* (Kinder, 1996). The aim was to provide realistic and effective HIV/AIDS education material dealing with unprotected anal sex within regular relationships for gay men. The social practice that had emerged from within the gay community was supported and endorsed.

Gay men knew that two HIV-negative men engaging in unprotected anal intercourse could not infect each other. The researchers who identified it (Kippax et al., 1993) understood that the specificities of gay men's sexual practice had important implications for HIV transmission and they too noted that unprotected anal intercourse was not necessarily unsafe. The argument advanced then and now is that dispensing with condoms is safe if the sexual partners are in a regular relationship, are HIV-antibody negative, are aware of each other's negative antibody status and have reached a clear and unambiguous agreement about the nature of their sexual practice both within and outside their relationship, such that any sexual practice outside their relationship is safe, that is, precludes the possibility of HIV transmission.

Evidence from Australia (Kippax et al., 1997; Crawford et al., 2001) and the Netherlands, which also endorsed negotiated safety as 'safe practice' (Davidovich et al., 2000), indicated that negotiated safety campaigns led to an increase in unprotected anal intercourse between regular partners, and these same studies have shown that the adoption of such a strategy did not lead to an increase in HIV transmissions in either country. In Australia, approximately one-third of gay men in regular relationships engage in this safe-sex practice (Jin et al., 2009). Although the proportion of men engaging in this practice has declined a little, it continues to be a practice understood and endorsed by the gay community (de Wit et al., 2014).

As biomedical developments were published and discussed within gay communities, other practices emerged in response to them. As noted in Chapter 3, these include 'strategic positioning', which is commonly used in serodiscordant relationships (Van de Ven, 2004) and, more recently, 'reliance on the undetectable viral load of one's HIV-positive partner' (Van de Ven, 2005). Practices have also emerged in conjunction with new technologies. For instance, Race (2015) describes the centrality of WIFI and 3G to the emergence of a very different form of sexual practice, 'party and play', among gay men. He demonstrates how online interactions are characterised by 'certain formal features that offer frameworks for constructing meaning and value' (255) that, in turn, give rise to various modes of sexual practice in the form of sexual play. The online interactions can include the pre-specification of particular sexual desires and activities as well as HIV status and viral load; sexual speculation and the co-construction of sexual fantasy; and the formation of what has come to be known as the 'extended session' or 'wired play' (267).

Other examples of similarly detailed accounts of the emergence of HIV-prevention responses in specific communities include, in Australia, among sex workers, Aboriginal Australians, people who inject drugs (Aggleton & Kippax, 2014); in the United States among gay men (Valdiserri, 2013) and people who inject drugs (Des Jarlais et al., 1995); and in Uganda and South Africa among networks of young people, workers and women (Thornton, 2008; Epstein, 2007); in Brazil (Paiva, 2003; Kippax et al., 2013;) and in Switzerland. (Dubois-Arber et al., 1999; Somaini, 2012). The accounts given in this research detail the emergence of community HIV-prevention strategies and associated social practices: such practices developed out of the social relations of the members of collectives.

In all these stories, and they differ from one another, there is reference to people coming together – as gay men, as young people, as sex workers, as people who inject drugs, as workers, as church goers, as HIV-positive women – each collective motivated to halt or reduce the spread of HIV within their communities. These accounts make little if any reference to any one individual, but rather to the strength or determination of the collective, typically aided by government funding and support. As discussed in Chapter 5, although the important role of collective agency in HIV prevention is mentioned by the Social Drivers Working Group, collective agency is cast as an aggregate of individual agency (aids2031 Social Drivers Working Group, 2010). The result is that the conceptual means to understanding modes of agency as they arise in *social relations* are overlooked. What is missing is how social practices and the norms that regulate them are produced by people acting together, in concert (Kippax, 2008), and it is to collectives, to communities, we now turn.

Community

There is a vital difference between the terms 'community' and 'group'. Epidemiological and biomedical discussion of 'groups', particularly 'risk groups', denotes something about aggregates of individuals without foregrounding that groups involve connections between people. Yet it is 'connectedness' between people and the glue that bonds them together, their engagement with one another, that is central – not only to the production of risk but importantly also to the production and fashioning of HIV-prevention strategies and the reduction of risk. Thus communities are not the abstracted 'risk groups' or 'populations' referred to by epidemiologists: they are not comprised of unconnected or isolated individuals. Communities or collectives of people are comprised of those who share (as well as contest and debate) understandings, beliefs, interests, activities and identities, and such communities have been, and continue to be, central to the effectiveness of HIV prevention.

Sociologists such as Clark (1973) have examined the multiple meanings of 'community': as locality, as identity, as solidarity. Although communities are often formed with reference to geographical location, in the context of the HIV epidemic, the notion of communities that hinge on 'identity' has obvious importance for HIV prevention: for example, gay men, people who inject drugs, 'young marrieds' – that is, those sub-populations identified by epidemiologists as 'at risk groups'. From the perspective of HIV prevention, what matters about these 'groups' is how they have formed and continue to form communities united by their interest in protecting themselves and their fellow community members. It is perhaps clearest with respect to the gay community, but it is also apparent in other affected communities, including sex workers, people who inject drugs, heterosexual men and women living in high-prevalence countries, people living with HIV and AIDS, and so on. Communities are formed on the basis of solidarity (Parker, 1996) and on the basis of shared sentiment and a desire to work together for the better good (Aggleton & Parker, 2015).

Communities play a number of roles in HIV transmission and prevention: they connect and engage people who have similar issues and concerns; they support the activities of people already involved in care and in HIV prevention, in drug treatment services and those already using sexual and reproductive health services; and they advocate and lobby with reference to HIV treatment and prevention. Effective public-health policies and HIV-prevention programmes build on a community sense of solidarity, common purpose and responsibility to fight HIV. Such fights in the form of responses to HIV take different paths because they emerge from communities and are of community. In the right circumstances, communities can enable and encourage dialogue and critical thinking and mobilise existing formal and informal networks, as well as build links with outside actors and agencies.[1] It is through such dialogue and action that social practices are modified and other practices, such as safe sex and safe drug injecting, are produced. Such community engagement shapes the norms that enable and sustain safe sex and safe drug use.

The social practices in which people engage co-constitute the world as it is, enabling communities to imagine, consider, discount, devise, adapt and adopt particular HIV-prevention strategies. This means that rather than trying to augment the capacities of individuals, effective prevention should focus on *the relations between people*, the norms that regulate such relations and the social practices that constitute them. As Williams (2003, 146) puts it, for HIV prevention to be effective, public-health practitioners need to understand people 'not simply [as] datum for epidemiological or sociological extraction' for the purpose of gauging 'risk' or 'vulnerability', but to understand how people relate to each other.

The Social Drivers Working Group foreground social research that recognises the community is central for social transformation. Vincent & Miskelly (2010), Campbell (2003, 2010) and Campbell et al. (2007), Auerbach et al. (2011), Seeley et al. (2012), Gibbs et al. (2012), Parkhurst (2012) and Schwartländer et al. (2011) all show the central role of community mobilisation and community participation. For example, Campbell (2010, 21) speaks of competence, as in 'AIDS-competent communities', arising to a large degree from facilitating 'programmes and processes that serve to buffer or ameliorate the impacts of social inequalities on people's health'. These researchers in various ways describe how communities, in connecting and engaging people, are central to the production of new social practices and the development of social norms.

Some, like Parkhurst (2012), conceptually align their research with the capability approach to social development advanced originally by Sen (1993, 2005). Parkhurst argues that rather than imposing a single goal or HIV-prevention strategy from outside, HIV programmes should build capabilities that enable people to achieve what *they* desire. For instance, gay men who affirm their identity as gay or who seek intimacy and pleasure in sexual activity have not embraced abstinence or foregone casual sex, but have devised a range of innovative sex-positive HIV prevention strategies and practices for minimising the risk of HIV transmission, many of which (for example, condom use) public health later adopted (Kippax & Race, 2003). A Social Drivers approach also points toward the key insights that can be drawn from the broader literature on social movements (Tarrow, 1996). These insights are important precisely because they emphasise how resistance to multiple forms of social inequality and exclusion can lead to the development of what Castells (1997), following Alain Touraine, has described as project identities – identities that produce and, in turn, are produced by broader collective projects aimed at social change in response to perceived inequities.

How communities transform social practices

In trying to interrogate *how* communities have the power to change and transform the social practices of their constituent members, others such as Thomas-Slayter & Fisher (2011) turn to the concept of social capital as developed in somewhat different ways by Bourdieu (1986) and by Putnam (2000). Researching social capital involves focusing on the social relations through which individuals or persons are embedded in their communities. It also leads to a focus on the resources of communities, such as information, knowledge, reputations and credits that 'flow through a set of social connections' (Thomas-Slayter & Fisher, 2011, 325) and to elucidating how particular communities emerge and the extent of their reach. Putnam (2000) and Woolcock (2001) distinguish three types of social capital evident in the relations between those in the community: bonding, bridging and linking. 'Bonding' refers to the relations between friends and family and, more generally, between people from the same demographic group. While also referring to horizontal ties between people, 'bridging' refers to ties that link or connect people from different demographic or spatial groups. 'Linking' social capital refers to a vertical trajectory that connects people across power structures. Viewed through the lens of social capital, Thomas-Slayter & Fisher (2011) concur with Campbell's (2009, 2010) characterisation of AIDS-competent communities as having the following characteristics:

1. The knowledge and skills to prevent HIV-transmission and [possessing] a means of translating their knowledge and skills into action in their own lives;
2. Social spaces for dialogue and critical thinking, so that people can collectively renegotiate individual and social norms that negatively impact the health and well-being of the community;
3. A sense of agency, [community] ownership and responsibility about the response to the epidemic;
4. A sense of solidarity and common purpose that allows people to work together despite potentially competing interests and to tackle the problem collectively;

5. Access to bridging and linking capital that provides the ability to connect with and access resources from outside communities or organisations that can support them in their efforts against the epidemic. (Thomas-Slayter & Fisher, 2011, 328–329)

As detailed in Chapters 2 and 3, the response of communities in Uganda and Australia – formed on the basis of solidarity as well as identity and locality – has clearly been central to the effectiveness of the countries' responses to HIV. Also, as discussed in Kippax et al. (2013), there are many other examples as demonstrated by studies of responses of countries and cities such as New York City, Rotterdam, Buenos Aries, Argentina and sites in Central Asia. Thomas-Slayter & Fisher (2011) discuss four case studies that demonstrate the effectiveness of HIV-prevention efforts premised on identifying and producing social capital within communities: in Andhra Pradesh in India, among female sex workers and men who have sex with men; in rural communities in South Africa; among female sex workers in the Kibera slum of Nairobi, Kenya; and in a multi-country study focusing on stigma reduction.

Other researchers give accounts of the importance of social network ties and associated communication patterns, such as documented by Friedman et al. (2007a, 2007b), in the Bushwick community in Brooklyn, New York. Meanwhile others speak of working in close participation with community members, such as in the initiatives of Stepping Stones in South Africa (Jewkes et al., 2008) and Avahan in India (Pickles et al., 2013). Further examples are also described in the publication of a special supplement of *AIDS Care* on the *Effects of Investing in Communities on HIV/AIDS Outcomes* (Rodrigues-Garcia, Wilson & York, 2013), in which community responses in Kenya, Benin, Nigeria, Zimbabwe, Lesotho and India have been evaluated. These studies provide rich and detailed accounts of the social and political processes involved in the collective shifts in social practices that preceded declining HIV incidence, and of the role of sexual communities, kinship networks, and drug using networks in achieving this outcome. It is demonstrable that collectives in the form of communities or networks are central in terms of advocating, initiating and implementing change via transformations in their social practices: 'The AIDS epidemic begins and ends in the community' (Simms, 2013, S1).

In Australia, for example, the importance of bonding, bridging and linking capital is evident in both the social and sexual engagement of gay men in the gay community (as discussed in Chapter 3) and the 'partnership' approach between communities, researchers, public health practitioners and government (Mindel & Kippax, 2013). In terms of resources, gay communities, people who inject drugs and sex workers were well-informed about modes of HIV prevention and reasonably well-resourced (although this is often subject to political contestation) to prevent transmission among the community and network members.

Affected communities and grass-roots activists also play a key role in shaping the social and political responses to HIV. Both Altman (1994) and Parker (2011), documenting the changing face of civil society in the response to HIV, point up the central role of grass-roots activists and affected communities. All around the world, people from a number of affected communities came together in order to help support and care for those with AIDS, to establish prevention programmes, to mobilise governments and to advocate for funding for treatment, care and prevention. By the mid-1980s NGOs committed to responding effectively to HIV and AIDS had emerged across the world. As Parker notes:

> It is impossible to overstate just how important grass roots pressure was – not only in industrialised countries in North America and Western Europe, but also in more resource-poor settings in Africa, Asia, Latin America and the Caribbean – in the push for recognition of the challenges posed by the epidemic and for protection of the rights of those affected by it. (2011, 24)

Brazil provides a clear example of the ways in which community mobilisation (among gay men as well as other marginalised groups) stimulated a broader social and political response (Parker, 1996). Community-based HIV prevention *later* provided the point of departure for the uptake of safe-sex approaches as part of official government programmes reaching wider populations. Perhaps because the HIV epidemic emerged during rapid political transformation with the return to democracy after a long military dictatorship, this political change at the national Brazilian level meant that there was considerable openness to early attempts to address the structural factors shaping the epidemic and the structural violence impacting the lives of affected communities. This led to a strong focus on resistance to social and economic oppression as key to government strategies aimed at responding to HIV and AIDS – and to the defence of human rights as a key part of HIV-prevention programmes (Daniel & Parker, 1993; Kippax et al., 2013).

In Brazil, an early focus, not just on identity, but also on solidarity between people affected by HIV in different ways led to the development of linkages across a range of diverse communities and populations. Gay, bisexual and other men who have sex with men, sex workers, and drug users were centrally important, but also quickly began to interface and collaborate with progressive religious organisations, labour unions, women's health and feminist organisations, youth groups and the emerging Black movement, among others (Berkman et al., 2005; Murray et. al., 2011). Solidarity emerged across a range of communities that perceived themselves to be vulnerable to the epidemic because of their shared status as historically marginalised and discriminated against; and this became the basis for a shared understanding of pushing back against the epidemic. AIDS activists in civil society and within the machinery of the state emphasised collective agency as an effective response to HIV and AIDS, building a rights-based strategy for HIV prevention as part of broader efforts aimed at ensuring the right to health (as articulated in Brazil's 1988 Constitution) as a fundamental part of citizenship (de Comargo, 2009). Perhaps the most important lesson from the Brazilian response to the epidemic has been its circumvention of individualistic prevention strategies and its focus on working toward structural change, a focus that is maintained without allowing the perception of structural obstacles to become a barrier to meaningful action. This coalition has gradually led to the development of one of the most progressive policy responses to the epidemic and to a wide range of prevention programmes implemented for and by many different communities (Nunn, 2009).

With reference to access to treatment, Parker (2011) provides another example of how community activism – in this case, by people living with HIV and AIDS – had extraordinary political success, globally. He describes how the political activity of NGOs in the global South has resulted in access to treatment for millions of people, particularly in countries where access to the new effective treatments was in the main limited to those who could afford it. Access to treatment became a priority among activists in the global South, and organisations such as TAC in South Africa and the Health GAP (Global Access Project) Coalition in the United States were established to fight for access for all to treatment. By 2002 a response to what had become a transnational treatment-access movement manifested itself in the Global Fund, the World Health Organization's (WHO) 3 x 5 programme, which aimed to provide antiretroviral treatment (ART) to 3 million people by 2005l; and a year later another significant actor entered the domain of treatment provision President's Emergency Plan for AIDS Relief (PEPFAR). As Parker (2011) notes, these developments would have been unimaginable even a decade earlier.

However as Seckinelgin (2008, 65) warns, some community or non-governmental organisations lose their connection to people, and '[t]here needs to be consideration of whether the link between people and attributed agency actually holds'. He points to examples from Botswana, Zambia and Rwanda demonstrating that the interventions implemented by community organisations reflected the policy interests of the international donors and organisations rather than the local and particular needs and interests of the community members. Seckinelgin (2008, 68) concludes: 'Most of these cases demonstrate a pattern where NGOs' assumed location within communities is used as a policy trope, while their links with people, that would have allowed different ways of thinking about interventions, are not valorised'. While NGOs are able to participate in international systems because of their links with people in the communities that those NGOs represent, this same participation runs the risk of dislocating them from their local communities. The critical perspectives of people in relation to their social worlds, their communities and institutions, are central to effective responses to HIV. Why such critical perspectives are lost in some cases and not in others is taken up in the final chapter, Chapter 7.

Conclusions

Notwithstanding the complexities, as indicated by Seckinelgin (2008), if there is one thing that the last 30 years of national and grass-roots experience in HIV have taught us, it is that communities and collective action provide the *possibilities* for change. Social change is always a function, not of individual behaviours, but of the collective actions and interactions of groups of people. Furthermore, social change is always emergent, often in response to the actions or omissions of others, such as when governments fail to act in relation to facilitating access to drug treatment or HIV prevention. Because such actions are contingent, social change is best understood as the unpredictable outcome of collective experimentation – experimentation that may work in unintended ways, such as when actions regarding HIV trigger broader education and health-sector reform (Race, 2012).

The argument we are making for understanding the malleable social practices that communities continually develop is animated by a body of work in the social sciences that attempts in different ways to address the limitations of notions of social structures as fixed and causal (Bourdieu, 1998). People act to transform the social via practices that they develop to respond to, in this case, HIV risk. In so doing, they transform the social. So-called macro structures are not literally out of reach, but they endure or transform to the extent that they can respond to and accommodate the demands arising out of the connections between people. Effective public health policies and HIV-prevention programmes build on a sense of solidarity, common purpose and collective responsibility to fight HIV and AIDS. The fight inevitably takes different paths and has different outcomes because it is the community and its members who build (in the sense of devise) and to some degree implement the response. In the right circumstances, communities can enable and encourage collective dialogue and critical thinking, and can mobilise existing formal and informal networks as well as build links with outside actors and agencies. It is through such dialogue that social practices are modified and other practices, such as safe sexual and drug injection practices, are produced. It is also through such community dialogue and common action that norms that enable and sustain safe sex and safe drug injection are built (Henderson et al., 2009; Kippax, 2012).

However, the history of HIV prevention, as revealed in much of the HIV/AIDS research literature and in WHO and UNAIDS documents, suggests that prevention has been increasingly positioned within the domain of biomedicine. This privileging of the biomedical has had a number of outcomes. Notwithstanding the talk of 'risk groups' (and in part because these 'groups' are cast as aggregates of individuals rather than entities to be understood in their own right), HIV prevention is increasingly focused on individuals rather than on collectives. This, in turn, means that the changes that are needed to prevent HIV transmission are understood as something that individuals are expected to achieve as a result of their rational thinking and action.

Social practices and the communities in which they are embedded are rendered invisible. In place of understanding and working with social relations, As Adam argues: 'HIV prevention messages and research paradigms [particularly those that derive from biomedicine] rely on and reinforce the "calculating, rational, self-interested subject and commercialised individualism that is increasingly constitutive of thought and conduct in private and public life" (Smart, 2003, 7) of advanced capitalist societies' (2005, 344). In contrast, it is possible to develop HIV-prevention efforts that acknowledge and work with how communities 'know and show allegiance to care and community when circumstances permit' (Adam, 2005, 345). The focus on the behaviour of individuals fails to recognise that the social transformation necessary for an effective and sustainable response to HIV is a function of social practices that are enabled and regulated by social norms, and that these are produced collectively by communities working together.

Furthermore, with the increasing emphasis on HIV testing, the turn to the clinic enables governments to avoid public discussion of sex (and drugs). Prevention as well as treatment and care are privatised – behind closed doors, so to speak. Social transformation is difficult if not impossible to achieve in the clinic. A public voice is needed. Moreover, although stigma and discrimination are recognised as problems in clinic-based counselling, gender and sexuality are left unpoliticised. Existing power relations – between men and women, heterosexual and homosexual, sex worker and client – remain unchallenged because clinical interactions do not target and provoke public discussion and debate in the way that community-based interventions can. Biomedicalisation is distorting HIV-prevention efforts. In many ways we, as social scientists, have failed to position the social and cultural aspects of HIV high on the agenda, although many of us have tried to trouble certain myths and moralistic responses around sexuality and have attempted to engage the biomedical in discussions about these and related matters. HIV prevention demands that social scientists engage with biomedical scientists and vice versa. Efforts to prevent HIV need to be understood as they are encountered in real life – as biological and material, as emotional and affective, and as social, collective and institutional.

In addition to highlighting the limitations of individualistic responses, recognising the central role that community mobilisation plays in shaping effective responses to the epidemic also calls attention to the ways in which communities are embedded in wider social and political contexts. HIV and responses to it occur within particular social contexts: the urban, the rural, the school, the workplace, the family and so forth (Seckinelgin, 2008, 41). These contexts cannot simply be reduced to or equated with abstract social determinants that organise social inequality. In a much more immediate sense, they are social and political processes that are constitutive of people's lived experience and, in some instances, enable social action and transformation, whereas in other instances they may provide equally powerful impediments to collective agency and community mobilisation (McAdam, McCarthy & Zaid, 1996). Social and political contexts matter, and it is the interaction between affected communities and the social and political processes in which they are enmeshed that creates the conditions that may favour the possibilities for social change (enabling conditions such as respect for diversity and the rights of citizenship), or alternatively, undermine collective agency (through prejudice, stigma, discrimination, and denial of rights and recognition) (Bell, 2011, Bell & Aggleton, 2012). This social approach, which elsewhere has been termed social public health (Kippax & Stephenson, 2012), moves beyond a reliance on individual capacities or social structures or drivers as separate entities and recognises that individual capacities are intimately tied to the enabling (or disabling) character of social norms, practices and institutions which, in turn, are understood to be transformed or modified by community mobilisation and social movements. Emphasising community mobilisation and social movements focuses attention on the centrality of collective agency to any process of meaningful change in response to HIV and AIDS, and highlights the reasons why grassroots activism has so often been more effective in responding to the epidemic than have formal public-health programmes or interventions. Importantly, because the potency of collective agency lies in communities' experimentation with developing and adapting different forms of social connectedness, public health cannot hope to understand this process of experimentation via a fixed blueprint or model. Furthermore, as Race (2012) points out, any attempt to harness it that focuses on the implementation of universal solutions necessarily misses the malleable and contingent details of specific social processes that make sense of an experiment's successes or failures. Processes of individual and social change are linked via the domain of social relations that people and communities cultivate. HIV prevention needs first to interrogate the specificities of these malleable social relations so that it may then develop approaches aimed at enabling communities and, indirectly, their individual members, to develop HIV risk-reduction strategies by changing their sexual and injection practices or adopting HIV-prevention technologies (or doing both).

In order to avert approximately two million new infections each year, prevention efforts need to be strengthened so that they are cognisant of wider social, political and economic contexts. Crucially, programmes must engage with the social meanings of sex and drugs, of pleasure and intimacy, and these changes must be practical and acceptable to local social and cultural norms and practices. For effective and sustained HIV prevention, the fight must be taken from the privacy of the clinic to the public domain. Prevention has worked and will continue to work if governments support communities in ways that make sense to those at risk rather than to powerful conservative minorities. For those working in the domain of health it is tempting to say that the answers lie in the wider social, political and economic arenas, and not only in health, and to engage so-called operational or implementation scientists to translate into action the interventions that public health has endorsed. In this demarcation the complexities of thinking about the effectiveness of prevention efforts in the real world become problems for implementation scientists to tackle by, for example, 'creating demand' for prevention strategies that seem promising to public health. Alternatively, there are those who invoke these wider domains and argue that because they are shaped by social structures imagined as 'macro', they are unchangeable. Perhaps it is this difficulty in recognising, conceiving of, imagining and working with social change as part of public health's *core* business that has contributed to a problematic shift in HIV prevention over the years. In general, now over thirty years since civil society and communities mobilised to combat HIV, community input appears to be decreasing – at least in its more direct confrontational form. The very active engagement with researchers, public health officials, clinicians, educators, lawyers and government officials that has been so extraordinarily beneficial with reference to both treatment and prevention has declined and changed. There is a need to re-engage with communities everywhere. As Schwartlander et al. (2011, 2035) noted: 'Community mobilization is essential for an HIV/AIDS response'. And this need was recognised in 2012 by UNAIDS in a report released in conjunction with the International AIDS Conference in Washington, D.C., entitled, 'Together We Will End AIDS'. In a section headed 'Transforming Societies', communities are placed centre stage: '[N]othing has ever happened in HIV that was not driven by the communities most impacted' (UNAIDS, 2012b, 61).

However, acknowledging and working with the specificities of social practice poses real challenges for those invested in developing and supporting effective global HIV-prevention strategies. One of the most significant of these arises when policymakers and funders seek to identify strategies that can be reproduced in different contexts or 'scaled-up', and when their efforts are animated by ideas about scientific certainty. As Race (2014a, 259) notes, once we acknowledge that social practice is, by definition, 'a meaningful and variable activity, scientists put themselves at risk of never being able to assume that they know, once and for all, or finally, what is going on'. Instead, abstracted notions of 'behaviour' 'unfold into a series of practical relations: conversations, exchanges, disputes, ruminations, contextualizations'. This, in turn, means that there is no ready position from which we can claim 'objective knowledge' of those practices being studied. It raises questions about how scientific knowledge can be developed and used when the 'object' of that knowledge – social practice – is not fixed, and entails understanding subjective, lived experience. We take these issues up in the concluding chapter.

Chapter 7

RESEARCHING SOCIAL CHANGE, WORKING WITH CONTINGENCY

The transmission of HIV is the direct outcome of particular sets or patterns of social and cultural practice – or, as was claimed early in the epidemic with reference to gay men, it is a function of 'lifestyle'. Patterns of social and cultural practice also give rise to diseases such as lung cancer (as caused by smoking) and diseases associated with obesity, such as heart disease and diabetes. Increases and decreases in incidence rates of these diseases are, to a greater or lesser extent, a function of social practices. While it is true that individuals may find it difficult to act and modify their practice so as to avoid or reduce their risk, collectively people can and have acted to do just that. People around the world have stopped smoking, many have reduced their weight, many have changed their sexual and drug injection practices, and many have lobbied governments and industry to implement regulation and changes to support them.

The reduction of HIV transmission is to a very large extent in the hands of collectives, the communities affected by HIV: it is these communities that have produced social practices that have reduced HIV transmission. This is particularly evident in those countries where governments have supported and funded communities to act and to develop 'AIDS competence'. Roy Anderson (2000) claimed at the International AIDS Conference in Durban that we know what works. And we continue to know what works. Effective prevention involves the sustained uptake of a range of social practices that reduce the likelihood of the transmission of HIV. We have discussed a number of these: the reduction in the number of one's sexual partners; the use of condoms (for sex) and sterile needles and syringes (for injecting); the uptake of pre-exposure prophylaxis (PrEP) among HIV-negative people and the uptake of antiretroviral treatments (ART) among those who are living with HIV; and male circumcision. As we have argued, whether these strategies are considered behavioural or biomedical, they all involve changes in practice, changes that are regulated by the norms and conventions of the social world in which those affected by HIV live and in which they have sex and inject drugs.

In Chapters 2 and 3 we detailed how communities in Uganda and Australia came together to reduce HIV transmission by transforming their sexual practices and, in Australia, also their injecting practices. They were successful – at least in the first decade or two. In Chapter 6 we also referred to many other studies that demonstrate similar successes by communities, such as those in Brazil. And in the countries hardest hit by HIV, those in southern Africa, surveillance suggests that something has been working. As documented in Chapter 1, with some exceptions, HIV incidence has been reduced. However, as we have pointed out, in many countries and particularly in high-income countries, there recently has been a stalling in HIV prevention, and in some countries increases in HIV incidence. What has gone awry?

It is our claim that the increasing biomedicalisation of HIV prevention as documented in Chapters 4 and 5 is part of the problem. The privileging of biomedicine and the concomitant individualising and privatising of prevention in the clinic have functioned to remove HIV prevention from the public domain and are increasingly rendering it invisible. Although the recent turn to the social 'drivers' of HIV transmission holds promise to re-socialise HIV prevention, it does not take us far enough in terms of engaging with the social as it is lived, grasped and sometimes modified by collectives and communities. By failing to give an adequate account of collective agency, the turn to 'social drivers' risks reification of social structures or mystifying the processes through which they change. As Seckinelgin (2008) cogently argues, many peer organisations and non-governmental organisations (NGOs) are in danger of losing their connections with communities from which they emerged, as many of their activities fail to engage with the experiences and lives of people they are understood to represent, which is, in turn, because of the organisational constraints associated with working with international agencies. These constraints arise in part because international policy frameworks tend to assume generalised social structures and generalised targets and risk groups: 'This process frustrates [the NGOs'] ability to respond to the needs articulated within local institutional processes and relationships' (Seckinelgin, 2008, 66). Instead of policy and action being designed to engage with local specificities, as Barnett & Whiteside (2006) note, they are directed from within a clinical–medical framework, and even non-clinical socio-economic and cultural aspects of people's lives are referenced to the biomedical. This biomedical approach is animated by a notion of a universal solution to HIV transmission, a problematic fantasy we discuss below with reference to one of its contemporary manifestations, treatment as prevention (TasP), and by the more chronically enduring misconception about what randomised controlled trials (RCTs) can and cannot provide regarding evidence of effective HIV prevention.

In Search of a Magic Bullet

In the search for a 'magic bullet', treatment has become prevention. Since the success of ART as treatment for HIV in late 1996, ART has increasingly been seen as not only *aiding* prevention but, more recently, *as* prevention. It has been successfully used in the prevention of mother-to-child transmission (PMTCT) and, more recently, in post-exposure prophylaxis (PEP) and PrEP for HIV-negative persons, although as discussed in Chapter 4, PrEP has not been shown to be efficacious in all population groups, and there are concerns with regard to disinhibition and the risk of resistance (*Lancet Infectious Diseases*, 2011). ART is now hailed as prevention, TasP: ART reduces the viral load of those taking it, thus making HIV-transmission to their HIV-negative sexual partners and those with whom they share injecting equipment far less likely. Below, we consider how, despite good reason for caution, TasP is being hailed as a 'magic bullet'.

This 'magic bullet' account of TasP is illustrated by a May, 2011 *Lancet* editorial titled 'HIV Treatment as Prevention – It Works', which was endorsed by Hillary Clinton at the 2012 International AIDS Conference held in Washington, stating that the world was well on the way to eradicating HIV. And in December 2014, *Time* magazine's Health section ran with the heading 'The End of AIDS' (echoing, for a wider audience, a vision many in biomedicine had been holding since 2012). Does TasP spell the 'end of the epidemic'? Or is it the case, as Paul Harkin, a counsellor heading up HIV services in a poor area of San Francisco, stated: 'It's a laudable goal, but I think the rhetoric should get toned down, because it's a disservice to the whole idea of prevention' (Park, *Time*, 2014). Here, we examine the chasm between the rhetoric around TasP and the evidence to date for its real world effectiveness. Our purpose is not principally to answer the question about effectiveness although, actually, we can say now that after interrogating all the evidence for TasP to date, the prospect of an AIDS-free era is not yet in sight. Rather, we want to show how this vision, which has seized the imagination of those involved in HIV prevention globally, is illustrative of the broader and concerted push for the biomedicalisation of prevention. We also offer a way forward.

Treatment as Prevention (TasP)

The first report demonstrating the effectiveness of TasP was based on an analysis of longitudinal data from a large cohort of serodiscordant couples in Uganda (Vernazza et al., 2008). The analysis demonstrated that under certain conditions treatment of HIV greatly reduces the risk of HIV transmission within cohabiting heterosexual serodiscordant couples: the HIV-positive person is adherent to treatment (ART) and is suffering from no other infection. Under these conditions, ART reduces the viral load to an undetectable level and thus reduces the likelihood of onward transmission to sexual partners to near zero. The analysis undertaken by Vernazza et al. (2008) resulted in a consensus statement issued by the Swiss Federal Commission for HIV/AIDS in 2008. At this point, the notion of treatment as a means of prevention was not widely embraced.

Myron Cohen et al. (2011), in their HPTN052 study (an RCT), confirmed the above finding for stable cohabiting heterosexual couples in serodiscordant relationships, and calculated that the *efficacy* of TasP was 96 per cent. Cohen's findings, taken together with earlier mathematical modelling (Granich et al., 2009), were hailed by many as heralding 'the end of the epidemic'. Claims were made about *population* impact, and there was an immediate call to roll out TasP, with the *Lancet* editorial (May 21, 2011, 1719) endorsing TasP as a population strategy. In other words, the claim was being made by many people (some very influential) that if a large proportion of people living with HIV were on treatment then HIV acquisition would decline and HIV would eventually disappear. While ART does indeed result in lowered transmission risk for *individual members of cohabiting couples*, is it likely to be an effective *population* strategy? As the findings of both studies focused on heterosexual discordant cohabiting couples, they should not be generalised. Indeed, it is important to note that people who acquired HIV during the HPTN052 study from someone other than their *cohabiting regular partner* were excluded from the calculation of efficacy. In total, of the 38 people infected during the trial, 28 were infected by their cohabiting partners (with one in the immediate ART group and 27 in the delayed ART group) and 10 were infected from outside the relationship (Cohen, McCauley & Gamble, 2012). If these 10 participants had been included, efficacy would be far lower, and caution is needed with regard to the ways in which the claim is made that treatment is prevention.

Furthermore, while the modelling of Granich et al. (2009) indicates that TasP could be effective in that it would radically reduce HIV transmission, other models – using different assumptions – do not (for example, Wilson et al., 2008; Mei et al., 2011; Garnett et al., 2012; Kretzschmar et al., 2012). As Garnett et al. (2012) discuss, modelling shows that the extent of a reduction in HIV transmission depends primarily on whether optimistic or pessimistic assumptions are made about the programmatic use of antiretrovirals, and state: 'Only the most extremely optimistic scenarios predict that treatment alone can halt the HIV pandemic, and even these assume that treatment enables reductions in sexual risk behaviour' (2012, 162).

There are problems in generalising from trial data to the real world. There is a conflation of efficacy with effectiveness, a conflation that appears to have been ignored. The study by Cohen et al. (2011) demonstrated the efficacy of TasP, while the analysis by Vernazza et al. (2008) provided *some* data pertinent to the 'effectiveness' of TasP. There is little doubt that TasP is highly efficacious: the Cohen (2011) study demonstrated that a large improvement in health outcomes was achieved in individuals in a research setting, in expert hands, under ideal circumstances (Aral & Peterman, 1999). However, there is a need to establish how effective TasP is at the population level, and to confirm or otherwise the analysis of Vernazza et al. (2008) by studying subgroups of populations other than (and different from) the cohabiting serodiscordant heterosexual couples in Uganda. The findings of the studies that followed the publication of the Swiss Consensus Statement (Vernazza et al., 2008) and the World Health Organization's modelling (Granich et al., 2009) focusing on population impact do not unequivocally demonstrate the effectiveness of TasP – that is, its impact in the real world in terms of lowering HIV incidence, under resource constraints, in entire populations, or in specified subgroups of a population (Aral & Peterman, 1999). Notwithstanding the pleas of Granich et al. (2010) for increased rates of HIV testing and early uptake of ART, as we discuss below, in some places the results demonstrate an impact – in other places not.

As mentioned, some studies have shown a decline in HIV incidence over time in association with widespread uptake of ART: a study in British Columbia, Canada, among people who inject drugs, which demonstrated a decline in HIV acquisition (Montaner et al., 2010); a study among homosexually active men in San Francisco by Das et al. (2010); and two more recent studies focused on cohabiting couples: one in KwaZulu-Natal (Tanser et al., 2013) in a very large population-based prospective cohort study, and a study in China (Jia et al., 2013).

However, with the above notable exceptions, in many communities and regions, as the number of people on ART has increased, there has been no concomitant decline in HIV acquisition – for example, among gay male populations in Australia (Wilson, 2012), New Zealand (Saxton et al., 2011), France (as reported in Wilson, 2012), Switzerland (van Sighem et al., 2012) and the United Kingdom and North America (van Griensven et al., 2009; Sullivan et al., 2009). In these countries, where there are very high rates of ART uptake and adherence, and where population viral load has been shown to have declined, there has been no decline in HIV acquisition. Indeed, in many of these countries, there have been increases in HIV acquisition.

There are a number of factors that appear to explain the differences between studies that show declines in HIV incidence associated with expansions in treatment uptake and those that find increases in HIV incidence. Not only may there be differences for different modes of transmission, but risk compensation or behavioural disinhibition may also account for the apparent ineffectiveness of ART as prevention. As noted by Fallon & Forrest (2012), and, as we have pointed out above, the efficacy of TasP demonstrated in the HPTN052 trial (Cohen et al., 2011) was calculated on the basis of *cohabiting* couples, most of whom were heterosexual. A very large proportion of gay men have multiple partners, and applying TasP to these communities that have much lower rates of monogamy is likely to result in 'unlinked' new infections (and these unlinked infections were excluded in the HPTN052 trial). As Holtgrave et al. (2012) have pointed out, some sub-populations of people living with HIV carry greater HIV-transmission risk than others. The interplay between serostatus discordance, risk behaviours and detectability of viral load differs. In Sydney, Australia, a recent study (Jin et al., 2010) has demonstrated that despite around 70 per cent of HIV-infected men being on antiviral treatment, and a high proportion of these men having an undetectable viral load,[1] the per-contact probability of HIV transmission due to unprotected anal intercourse is similar to estimates reported from the income rich world in the pre-ART era. That is, it is possible that treatment is not as effective in reducing infectiousness in gay male populations because the per-contact probability of HIV transmission via anal intercourse is ten-fold higher than by vaginal intercourse, because of the higher rates of sexually transmissible infections in gay male populations, and because of risk compensation and the associated decline in condom use by gay men (Wilson, 2012). Regarding risk compensation, there is evidence from behavioural surveillance in Australia that unprotected anal intercourse with casual sexual partners is increasing (as discussed in Chapter 3). Socio-behavioural studies in Australia (Zablotska et al., 2009; Bavington et al., 2013) have also shown risk compensation among gay men: with gay men with undetectable viral load (and their partners) more likely to engage in unprotected anal intercourse than those with detectable viral load.

With regard to the four studies cited above that demonstrate an association between TasP and a decline in HIV incidence: there has been some caution expressed about interpreting the results of the Canadian study (Montaner et al., 2010) and the study in San Francisco (Das et al., 2010) as evidence for the success of TasP. The timing of the Montaner et al. study is pertinent for interpreting their results; there had recently been a large intervention among people who inject drugs, which some believe may account for the decline in HIV transmission. More importantly, no risk compensation is likely among people who inject drugs. Unlike condoms, which are not necessary for sexual engagement, not only are needles and syringes required to inject, it is in people's interest to use clean needles: fewer abscesses, less bruising, better injecting experience, less risk of Hep C transmission, etc. With regard to the 2010 San Francisco study, Garnett et al. (2012) note that the 'positive result' may be due to other factors, and that one would 'expect a delay between incident infection and an infectious case being diagnosed and reported' (160).

The two more recent studies, cited above, conducted in China (Jia et al., 2013) and in Hlabisa, KwaZulu-Natal (Tanser et al., 2013) demonstrated a significant and strong relationship between ART coverage and reduction in HIV acquisition. However, it is important to note that although Jia et al. (2013) confirm the effectiveness of TasP with reference to serodiscordant couples (their study based on 38,862 serodiscordant couples showed a 26 per cent reduction in HIV transmission under real-world conditions), they note that 'protection was only significant in the first year' (6). They are unsure of the reasons for this and comment that the *long-term* durability of the protectiveness of treatment needs to be confirmed in additional studies.

In Hlabisa, which comprises around 60,000 people who were participants in the open population cohort, about 80 per cent consented to be tested for HIV. ART coverage rose from 10 per cent to 30–40 per cent of all HIV-infected individuals over a six-year period. Given this proportion of people on ART is not high when compared with that in Australia and many countries in Western Europe, why the strong and very positive finding? Barnighausen (2013, personal communication) has suggested that in settings such as rural KwaZulu-Natal, where increased access to ART has transformed the community life: many people living with HIV have been able to go back to work and lead normal lives, and renewed hope has meant that they take more care now regarding HIV transmission. Indeed the study (Tanser et al., 2013) reported a significant increase in condom use among regular partners in the years between 2005 and 2011, which was independent of the strong relationship between ART coverage and the lowered risk of HIV acquisition. This study clearly demonstrates evidence for the effectiveness of TasP in this setting as well as the absence of any behavioural disinhibition or risk compensation or, indeed, the presence of what might be called 'risk-reduction enhancement'. It is possible, as Wilson (2012) has suggested, that ART may have less impact in reducing new HIV infections in countries or among populations where very high levels of ART coverage have been reached, as in Europe and Australia – a sort of ceiling effect.

Many researchers have commented on these and other studies. Wilson (2012) sums up, saying that the examination of data from treatment as prevention 'natural experiments' suggests there are limitations to reductions in population HIV incidence. He points to limitations in terms of risk compensation, difficulties in linking people living with HIV to treatment and retaining them in clinical care, and the increasing pool of potential transmitters produced by successful ART. In a similar way, Mei et al. (2011), with reference to men who have sex with men in Amsterdam, point to problems in risk compensation and

argue that lowering risk behaviour is the most important population prevention measure – even in the presence of TasP.

To these more cautious considerations of the reach and limits of TasP we
would add that, if TasP leads to an anchoring of HIV-prevention efforts in the
clinic, then there is a real risk that it will function to further privatise HIV, making HIV (whether we are talking about treatment or prevention) a matter for
individuals or couples, and not for broad public discussion, debate and action.
We have seen (for example, in Chapter 2, in discussing the rise, fall and then
rise of HIV incidence in Uganda) how central collective, public involvement is
to the response to HIV in reducing incidence, and how (for example, in discussing HIV testing in Chapter 5) clinic-based responses can function to position
people as patients or information recipients, rather than engaging them in collective attempts to devise and develop apt responses to transmission.

Although there are few in biomedicine or, indeed, in social science who doubt
the *efficacy* of TasP and its value to the HIV-negative partner living in a serodiscordant relationship,[2] what these studies demonstrate is that TasP may be effective at the population level *only* under *certain conditions* and *only* in *certain contexts*;
not exactly a 'magic bullet'. Cohen et al. (2012) and Muessig & Cohen (2014)
acknowledge the differences and note: 'Implementation of ART as prevention
faces substantial challenges, including logistical limitations, potential challenges
in risk-taking behaviors, and cost' (Cohen et al., 2012, 1594). However, they
seem to think that there is a 'best strategy' for the use of antiretrovirals, one
that has not yet been developed (1585). As social scientists we would argue that
there is unlikely to be a 'best strategy' because the reasons for the differences
between the studies lie in the social and cultural differences in the populations
under study: the effectiveness of any HIV-prevention strategy is the *contingent*
outcome of the collective activity of a diverse range of actors, both human
and non-human, including the mode of prevention being adopted, scientific
practices, clinical services, cultural, political and social environments, and the
norms, values and discourses that animate human behaviour or practice (Race,
2012). There is no 'best strategy': even in one specific context the effectiveness
of any particular prevention strategy is likely to change over time, particularly
as there are new developments in the field of HIV and in communities' understanding of and access to treatment and different means of prevention. Effectiveness of a strategy does not simply depend upon how well an efficacious
HIV-prevention 'technology' is implemented.

Working with *All* the Evidence

Ensuring that people take up efficacious prevention strategies – whether one
is speaking of condoms or ART – is not simply a matter of 'implementation'

scientists' implementing the 'proven' HIV prevention technologies and pro-grammes. Rather, what is required, as noted at the end of the previous chapter and the beginning of this, is the genuine engagement of communities, particu-larly those communities at risk of HIV. Community engagement is required not only with the delivery and uptake of prevention, but with the delibera-tion and design of particular prevention strategies. Particular communities will produce particular responses, including risk-reduction strategies that are acceptable to them – a fact entirely missed by a focus on 'implementation science'.

However, with the increasing medicalisation of HIV prevention, the mobil-isation of communities, recognised as central to HIV prevention by Schwartz-lander et al. (2011) and UNAIDS (2012c), has been undermined and in some ways perverted. Instead of engaging with communities and understanding their practices, implementation scientists seek instead to address the 'barriers' to effective implementation of pre-established strategies. For example, Sturke et al. (2014, S163) define implementation science as 'an approach which aims to investigate and address major bottle-necks that impede effective implemen-tation of scientifically proven interventions for public health impact and to test new approaches to identifying, understanding, and overcoming barriers to the implementation of these interventions'. However, social and cultural prac-tices are not bottlenecks or barriers that 'impede effective implementation' and that need to be 'overcome'. These so-called barriers are the stuff of com-munities: they are the social practices of the communities and the norms that regulate those practices. Because HIV is transmitted by some of these prac-tices, they also can provide the way forward to the eradication of HIV. Genu-ine community engagement is indispensable to HIV prevention. Yet Sturke et al. (2014, S163) state that advancing implementation science will require efforts to facilitate 'collaboration, communication, and relationship-building among researchers, implementers, and policy makers'. Note the absence of 'community' here. Although later on in their paper, Sturke et al. (2014, S166) mention the need to include 'representatives from HIV-affected communi-ties', the overall sense of implementation science is that HIV interventions, programmes and messages come from the top down – from the expert to the individual. There is no discussion of how to ensure community involvement and commitment.

With reference to a large number of examples, Seckinelgin (2008, 68) notes that positioning prevention as a matter of 'implementation' has the effect that 'NGOs gradually become dissociated from their social spaces. In the eyes of the people they become actors of international interventions rather than long-term partners for change'. The 'representatives from HIV-affected com-munities' referred to by Sturke et al. (2014) fail to find points where their communities and the community members' perspectives can be actively put to work in shaping the decisions and actions of the institutions charged with HIV prevention. TasP and the associated increase in biomedicalisation are likely to exacerbate this problem with policies increasingly targeting people who are HIV-positive and understood first and foremost as 'patients'.

What this means in the context of TasP, which Seckinelgin appears to have anticipated, is that:

> [p]eople living with the disease in diverse socio-economic and cultural contexts are transformed into target populations living with HIV/AIDS. Most contextual differences are ignored by focusing on the existence of the HIV virus in individual bodies. This move allows international actors to devise generalised abstract policies to help these target populations or risk groups. However people's experiences of both the disease and the policies demonstrate that there is a considerable gap between this approach and the way people live with the disease. Since international actors are not sensitive to the way people live and the implications of the disease in their everyday lives, policies target more and more what are seen as patient populations or risk groups. (2008, 147)

In many cases, engagement with community has been reduced to token membership of a 'representative' on international public health committees. The notion of collective agency and the social, economic and political realities of people's lives are lost in the search for 'scientifically proven' suit-all HIV-prevention strategies with little if any understanding of the contingent nature of effectiveness. Efficacy and effectiveness are conflated. It seems that once the 'efficacy' of an HIV-prevention technology is demonstrated, it becomes the job of implementers to ensure its 'rollout', overcoming the so-called social barriers and bottlenecks.

The insistence on 'scientifically proven' interventions, where 'scientifically proven' is understood to mean demonstrated by RCTs or at the very least experiment, helps explain why the Swiss Consensus Statement (Vernazza et al., 2008) was greeted by many with disquiet, while the HPTN052 trial of Cohen et al. (2011) was hailed. As Jon Cohen (2011, 1628) recounts in his commentary of TasP published in the journal *Science*, the publication of the Swiss Statement was denounced by many as 'appalling', 'inconclusive and irresponsible', 'dangerous' and 'misleading' and the 'Joint United Nations Programme on HIV/AIDS and the World Health Organization also responded with alarm'. However, as he goes on to note with regard to the HPTN052 trial: '[N]ow a growing number of HIV/AIDS experts are insisting that the irresponsible and appalling thing to do is nothing' (1628). So taken was the biomedical world with the findings of the Myron Cohen et al. (2011) study – an

RCT – that the earlier Swiss Consensus Statement is commonly forgotten. In part the reason for this strange outcome is that many in biomedicine (for example, Padian et al., 2010) have argued that RCTs are necessary to demonstrate effectiveness. Furthermore, many in international NGOs and agencies have accepted this argument (for example, Mburu et al., 2014) and have concluded: 'Until recently, HIV prevention lacked credibility with data from prevention trials showing little or no decrease in incidence of HIV/AIDS' (40). The insistence on experiments has also led many working in HIV to doubt the real-world impact of many HIV-prevention programmes that relied on condom use and other changes in social practice (as discussed in Chapter 1). This narrow and problematically limiting approach to 'evidence' is illustrated by the *Lancet* editorial's (2011, 1719) argument that funding agencies such as the President's Emergency Plan For AIDS Relief and the Global Fund to Fight AIDS, Tuberculosis and Malaria 'need to reassess their prevention portfolios and consider diverting funds from programmes with poor evidence (such as behavioural change communication) to treatment for prevention'. It is disquieting that influential journals, such as the *Lancet* call on HIV-prevention experts not to waste money on behavioural change communication. As social scientists 'looking on', we are left wondering about the valorisation of the findings of RCTs and the lack of understanding regarding the particularity and fluidity of effectiveness.

This problematic emphasis on RCTs is evident in patterns of the National Institutes of Health (NIH) funding of HIV-prevention research. Green & Kolar (2014) demonstrate the impact of holding up RCTs as the gold standard of prevention research by comparing studies designed to elucidate risk-taking with studies proposing to evaluate the 'efficacy' of interventions. Between 2001 and 2012 only 8 per cent of funded intervention studies took a 'strong' social-science approach, that is, 'mak[ing] interpretive and structural contexts central to the focus of research, rather than an "add-on" to an otherwise biomedical individualist research project' (2014, 6). Fifty-five per cent of funded intervention studies took an entirely biomedical individualistic approach, and another 28 per cent were largely biomedical in approach but included a component (either weak or moderate in terms of its integration into the grant as a whole) that involved trying to address the meanings or the social structures pertinent to HIV prevention.[3] In a sense, this is evidence of something that is already well known. However Green & Kolar's (2014) research indicates a striking internal contradiction within the funding of HIV-prevention research by the NIH. Looking at research designed to elucidate risk-taking, again funded between 2001 and 2012, only 7 per cent was marked by a biomedical individualist framing – with a further 25 per cent being biomedical with some weak or moderate social component. A strong interpretative and structural approach was evident in 27 per cent of the funded grants. This suggests that, within this scientific community, there is some acceptance of the need to understand risk in the social contexts in which it arises (more than a quarter of their funding is allocated to it), but that this knowledge is failing to translate into the funding of interventions. Why is it that research that contributes to knowledge of HIV transmission risk is not being put to work in the way that is intended and funded to do, that is, by informing interventions that aim to reduce risk? The answer given by Green & Kolar (2014) is that the notion of RCTs as the gold standard of research is not as widely shared by researchers producing knowledge of risk as it is in the domain of intervention research.

However, the epistemological difference between the disciplines of the social and the biomedical sciences is a more radical one. Interventions cannot be evaluated by RCTs because the manner in which interventions are responded to – whether they are taken up, rejected, modified, forgotten, misunderstood, sustained, and so on – is the outcome of social processes. To assume that somehow the efficacy of an intervention (as opposed to the efficacy of a prevention technology) can be evaluated independently of its effectiveness in the real world is to commit a category error (Kippax, 2003).

Furthermore, as argued by Kippax (2003), Parkhurst (2008) and McMichael & Rosengarten (2013), such insistence on RCTs to establish prevention effectiveness is quite inappropriate and has done much damage, for example, leading many to believe that earlier prevention efforts have failed. The evidence required for effectiveness is population health improvement – in the case of HIV, a decline in HIV incidence – gathered over time in the real world (as discussed in Chapter 4). With regard to TasP, as has been shown above, effectiveness has not been consistently found. While the evaluation of the efficacy of a prevention technology is typically demonstrated using RCTs or experiment and can be generalised to all populations under all conditions, or so it is usually assumed,[4] the evaluation of effectiveness requires evidence over the long term of the particular strategy's adoption and sustained use, in the absence of any risk compensation or disinhibition. Phase IV trials are needed to establish effectiveness, or research of the type that Vernazza et al. (2008) provided in their analysis of long-term cohort data. Public health needs to know how and in what ways particular social, political and economic conditions influence the take-up and sustained use of HIV prevention strategies by communities.

Paradigms: Biomedical and Social

The major problem that this book has addressed and attempted to respond to is related to the two very different ways of understanding and doing HIV prevention: the biomedical and the social.

From the standpoint of biomedicine, a very important part of the work of biomedical researchers is to develop efficacious 'HIV-prevention technologies'. Public health's role is to ensure that the efficacious technologies are adopted and their use sustained in people living with HIV and in populations deemed at risk of HIV infection. It is not difficult to understand the appeal of the biomedical paradigm, and there is no doubt that prophylaxis in the form of oral drugs such as PrEP could be – at least for many people – easier to incorporate into everyday life than abstaining from sex, reducing numbers of partners or using condoms. However a strategy such as PrEP is not without its difficulties: there are a number of problems over and above those identified by biomedical researchers such as Cohen et al. (2012), including resistance, long-term biological effects and adherence. For example, with reference to serodiscordant couples in the United States, McMahon et al. (2014) raise questions around cost, risk compensation[5] and acceptability. Further, although some individuals may find PrEP acceptable, there is concern, for example, among sex workers in Australia (personal communication), that PrEP will undermine the extremely effective HIV-prevention response of close to 100 per cent condom use by clients, and that pressure will be placed on sex workers to use PrEP (Bates & Berg, 2014).

Within the biomedical/public health paradigm, populations are understood to be comprised of unconnected individuals, and these individuals are understood to be neo-liberal subjects, who have agency and respond rationally to the authority of public health. It is assumed that if given the information with regard to HIV transmission, they – in the absence of 'barriers' – will do as asked and get tested, refrain from unsafe behaviours and adopt HIV-prevention technologies such as condoms, microbicides and, if HIV-negative, male circumcision and PrEP, and if HIV-positive, initiate treatment early to aid in HIV-prevention. The provision of information about prevention, the intervention, has increasingly been positioned as happening in the clinic – as the counselling that attends testing. There have also been references to communication, such as school education and forms of mass communication, but the 'implementation' of HIV-prevention interventions is mainly imagined as the designated task of 'implementation scientists' who, it is assumed, will somehow or other 'create a demand for' the latest HIV-prevention technology.[6] However, the primary lesson that can be drawn from the findings of Niang & Boiro (2007) with reference to the promotion of male circumcision is that efforts to 'create a demand' should move quickly beyond the narrow realm of biomedical intervention to engage with socio-cultural meanings and practices. And, we would add, the same applies to all biomedical interventions.

As discussed above, although the importance of community is acknowledged, community engagement is typically reduced to a community representative or two on clinical trials. Furthermore, as discussed above, the interventions are increasingly top-down, with public health positioned as the authority. Although biomedical and public health researchers recognise that economic, political and social factors may make it difficult for individuals to act appropriately, that is, rationally, they tend to understand such social and other factors as barriers. As a result, their responses to social and economic factors such as gender and poverty have been to tackle such inequalities by, for example, financing high school education for some girls. As discussed in Chapter 5, such interventions do nothing to change the ways in which schools reinforce gender inequalities (Gibbs et al., 2012), that is, the social practices through which gender inequalities are produced, reproduced and may or may not change are left in a 'black box' rather than interrogated. Other structural interventions seek to circumvent social and political factors by, for example, advocating the use of PrEP in countries that are unwilling to establish needle and syringe programmes for people who inject drugs, as in Thailand. Because the research and related policy proceed from an understanding of the social, economic and political informed by the biomedical paradigm, such interventions are typically 'top-down' and are unlikely to succeed – even in the short term.

The biomedical paradigm is one that makes sense in the contexts of treatment and, indeed, for HIV prevention, if an efficacious vaccine were available. However, it is unable to address the wider social issues that are currently central to an effective HIV-prevention response: issues related to social practices and normative regulation, and to community engagement. Although there is talk of 'combination prevention', where the term is meant to convey that what is needed is a combination of biomedical, behavioural and structural interventions, the term at present has only rhetorical significance. There is a belief that once efficacious 'technologies' are provided, they will be effective HIV-prevention strategies for all peoples and populations. As Nguyen et al. (2011, 291) note in their opinion piece in the journal *AIDS*, there has been a 'striking remedicalisation of our approach to the HIV epidemic and a return to the early 1980s view of the epidemic as a medical problem best addressed by purely technical, biomedical solutions whose management should be left to biomedical professionals and scientists'.

From the standpoint of *social science*, a very important part of the work of social scientists is to engage with communities, networks and other collectives to ensure that efficacious HIV-prevention strategies are adopted and their use sustained. In other words, their major task is to enable communities to protect themselves from HIV and so reduce HIV transmission and, in the long term, reduce HIV incidence. Their focus is the local and particular – rather than on universal solutions. The work of social scientists is needed in tandem with that of biomedical scientists.

The social paradigm focuses on the relations between people, the norms that regulate such relations and the social practices that constitute them. The individual, the person, is understood as a social being. The approach moves beyond a reliance on individual capacities and attempts to understand the ways in which groups and communities as well as institutions respond to outside threats, such as HIV. It is also distinct from taking social structures or drivers as one's entry point into HIV prevention. The social paradigm allows us to see how social norms enable (or hinder) individuals' actions – reproducing social practices and occasionally producing new social practices via community mobilisation and social movements. Processes of individual and social change are linked and, within the social sciences, HIV prevention is understood in terms of enabling communities and, indirectly, their individual members, to develop HIV risk-reduction strategies by changing their sexual and injection practices or by adopting HIV-prevention strategies. As Gibbs et al. (2012) argue, it is essential to work closely with organisations that have local, contextual or insider knowledge.

Mechanisms that enable a collective response to HIV are not the outcome of one or more particular formal health communication or HIV-prevention intervention. Rather, social mobilisation via public discussion and talk triggers shifts in the social norms shaping the meaning of sexual relationships and sexual and injecting practices. The approach typically focuses on how peers (including opinion leaders) engage with one another and how they, *together*, change their practices to reduce HIV transmission without foregoing pleasure and desire. The communication is horizontal rather than top-down.

Effective public health policies and HIV-prevention programmes build on a sense of solidarity, common purpose and collective responsibility to fight HIV and AIDS. The fight inevitably takes various paths and involves various outcomes because it is the community and its members who build, in the sense of devise, and to some degree implement, the responses. In the right circumstances, communities can enable and encourage collective dialogue and critical thinking, and mobilise existing formal and informal networks as well as build links with outside actors and agencies. It is through such dialogue that social practices are modified and other practices, such as safe sexual and drug injection practices, are produced. It is also through such community dialogue and common action that norms that enable and sustain safe sex and safe drug injection are built. Recognising the central role that community mobilisation plays in shaping effective responses to the epidemic also calls attention to the ways in which communities are embedded in wider social and political contexts. These contexts cannot simply be reduced to or equated with abstract social determinants that organise social inequality; in a much more immediate sense, they are social and political processes that in some instances enable social action and transformation, whereas in other instances they may provide equally powerful impediments to collective agency and community mobilisation (Kippax et al., 2013, 1373).

Social and political contexts matter, and it is the interaction between affected communities and the social and political processes in which they are enmeshed that creates the conditions that may favour the possibilities for social change (enabling conditions such as respect for diversity and the rights of citizenship), or alternatively, may undermine collective agency (through prejudice, stigma, discrimination and denial of rights and recognition).

This social approach, which elsewhere has been termed a social public health (Kippax & Stephenson, 2012), moves beyond reliance on individual capacities or social structures or drivers as separate entities, and recognises that individual capacities are intimately tied to the enabling (or disabling) character of social norms, practices and institutions, which are, in turn, understood to be transformed or modified by community mobilisation and social movements. This emphasis on community mobilisation and social movements focuses attention on the centrality of collective agency to any process of meaningful change in response to HIV and AIDS, and it highlights the reasons why grassroots activism has so often been more effective in responding to the epidemic than have formal public health programmes or interventions. Importantly, because the potency of collective agency lies in communities' experimentation with developing and adapting different forms of social connectedness, public health cannot hope to understand this process of experimentation via a fixed blueprint or model. Furthermore, as Race (2012) points out, any attempt to harness collective agency that focuses on the implementation of universal solutions necessarily misses the malleable and contingent details of specific social processes and forces that make sense of an experiment's successes or failures. Processes of individual and social change are linked via the domain of social relations that people and communities cultivate. HIV prevention needs first to interrogate the specificities of these malleable social relations so that it may then develop approaches aimed at enabling communities (and, indirectly, their individual members) to adopt HIV-prevention strategies and, where necessary, to change their sexual and injection practices.

Working Together

There is no doubt that HIV is a medical condition. However HIV being a medical condition does not in itself change the social relationships and institutions affecting its transmission or its consequences. Nor does it mean that the social can be subsumed in attempts to enable effective HIV-prevention responses or that people can be abstracted from their social worlds and local knowledge systems (Seckinelgin, 2008, 76). Rather an effective HIV prevention response requires multidisciplinary teams – teams in which community members, social scientists and biomedical scientists have equal footing. Community members know what it is like to be a drug user, a gay man, a sex worker, an HIV-positive person and so on. Vico ([1725] 2002), the eighteenth-century Italian philosopher, argued that 'the true is the made'. Understanding something from an outsider's perspective is one form of knowledge, and another form of understanding is 'what it is like to be' or 'what it is like to do' – that is, knowledge stems from enactment in practice. This is not to discount what outside, or expert, perspectives can bring to understanding an HIV epidemic, but to make clear that the knowledge of those who are experiencing, acting on and in an epidemic is invaluable to effective HIV-prevention programmes because the practices of community members, the practices that people produce are the building blocks of effective HIV-prevention responses.

We have said much in this book about people's social practices – HIV prevention involves the practices that produce, reproduce and transform the social worlds in which people live. As scientists we need to have knowledge of the forces shaping the epidemic – whether social, structural, geographic, historical, political or economic – and their connection to those practices. Social practices (sexual and drug injection practices) are complex and fluid processes. In order to fully grasp and understand them, we need to see the world from the point of view of the community members who enact them as well as from our own positions as social or political or biomedical scientists (Stephenson & Kippax, 1999; Kippax & Stephenson, 2005; Stephenson & Kippax, 2006). If we do not do this the evidence we claim will at best always be partial.

We need to acknowledge that there are different ways of 'doing science' or knowing, and we need to listen to those who practice 'sex' and 'drug use' in the variety of ways in which these processes (or objects of science) are engaged. If as scientists we artificially fix these complex objects via our attempts to produce definitive knowledge, then we are likely to lose the active participation of community members and, hence, fail to grasp the ways in which they define the problems of HIV and can devise effective responses to them (Rosengarten, 2009). Indeed, Race (2016) claims that community has already been disengaged from research and policy areas. Race argues that a 'tacit commitment' of HIV prevention 'is to manage and flatten the affective intensities, complications, and disturbances of sex' (2012, 7). Because of this, HIV prevention, regardless of the rhetoric or scientific justification accompanying it, cannot do otherwise than interrupt notions of science that are based on regulatory distinctions between subject and object, private and public, the empirical and the speculative, rationality and affect. In other words in studying sex and drug use, we, as scientists, must not require our research participants or indeed community members to disavow their own immersion in sexual (and drug) cultures and forms of pleasure.

Unlike behaviour, practices are not fixed and cannot definitively be extracted from contexts, isolated and measured. Practice is central to our devising, as community members and scientists, effective HIV-prevention responses – responses that will change from region to region, from community to community, from social context to social context, and over time. Efforts to prevent HIV are essentially efforts to change society. Notwithstanding the latest biomedical advances, there is no 'magic bullet'. With the development of HIV-prevention strategies, social and biomedical scientists together need to work with communities and *Acknowledge* difference, *Be* realistic and support *Collective* action – a far more acceptable and effective ABC.

NOTES

1. Mapping a Social Disease

1 Note, in the following account of regional and country epidemics, unless otherwise referenced all figures are taken from 2014 country reporting to UNAIDS (UNAIDS, 2014b).

2 This early high HIV incidence is likely to have been a function of the number of travellers to international organisations and meetings, many from Africa, before HIV was identified.

2. 'Owning' Uganda

1 Uganda Ministry of Health and UNAIDS researchers, Asiimwe-Okiror et al. (1997), provide further indications of declining prevalence from sentinel surveillance data in pregnant women in two urban districts. Between 1989 and 1996 prevalence rose and then dropped, with an overall decline of 40%. Although some sentinel surveillance in pregnant women in rural areas did not indicate the same marked decline, there were some similar findings in rural cohort studies (e.g., in Rakai, HIV prevalence in 13–24-year-olds dropped to 12.6% from 17.3% between 1990 and 1992 and, in Masaka, prevalence in 13–24-year-olds dropped from 3.5% to 1% between 1989 and 1994.

2 For example, in South Africa in 1988, 14% of people reported knowing someone with AIDS.

3 Rather than conclude that Lady Museveni's performance was the result of the new imposition of a foreign ideology, it needs to be remembered that from the outset the Ugandan public health response was distinguished by the myriad international funders and actors involved at all levels from technical expertise through to NGO involvement at the local level (e.g., WHO, WHO-AFRO, the World Bank, international NGOs). The 'home-grown' Ugandan public health approach to HIV prevention was a massive social experiment involving alliances between these international agencies and Ugandan agencies and decentralised actors who – for a short time – aligned with the social terrain that Ugandans had cultivated in the late 1980s and enabled HIV prevention in the form of open discussion.

4 In addition to the problematic neglect of 'C', the conflation of the strategy 'reduction of number of sexual partners' with the strategy 'B' or monogamy, as we will show below, has very serious consequences for HIV transmission. While reduction in the number of sexual partners clearly limits HIV transmission, if one's sexual partner is of a different HIV status, monogamy is not a safe sexual strategy.

5 DHS (the figure was not reported in 2006). The trend is in the reverse for men, with 58% of men against the idea in 2000–2001 and only 34.3% against it in 2011.

6 Primary school education was made free in 1997; in 2005 Cohen & Tate noted that in many rural schools a high proportion of students were in their teens as they were taking up this opportunity.

7 From the 2010 country report: 'Initially, condoms were not heavily promoted and distributed during the early years of the AIDS epidemic in Uganda, as they were considered to offer false hope that the epidemic could be stopped without curbing multiple sexual partnerships. This changed in [the] mid-1990s when condoms were widely distributed, raising the number delivered and promoted by international groups from 1.5 million in 1992 to nearly 10 million in 1996. About 130.7 million condoms were procured and distributed by MoH, MSI, PSI (now PACE) and AFFORD as compared with 107.5 in 2006 or 39.1 [million] in 2004. During 2008–2009, the government received condom procurement support from organisations, mainly UNFPA, AHF Uganda Cares, AMREF and Marie Stopes International. Messages on condom use have been passed using print and broadcast media. Many billboards and posters have messages such as "use a condom correctly and consistently"' (38).

8 If we infer that the same gap between knowledge and actual access holds true today as it did in 2000–2001 the percentage of young women (15–24 years) who think that they can actually access condoms would be around 57%.

3. The Australian Partnership

1 It was not the case that those gay men who knew people with HIV or had known people who had died of AIDS were any more or less likely to adopt safe sex and use condoms than gay men who did not know people with HIV, had nursed people with AIDS or had known people who had died. Contact with the epidemic (the scale that was composed of these three items) was not associated with men adopting safe sex in 1986–1987 (Kippax, Connell, Dowsett & Crawford, 1993) – whereas contact with the community was.

2 However, it is important to note that people who acquired HIV during this study from someone other than their *cohabiting regular partner* were excluded from the calculation of efficacy. This and related issues are addressed in Chapters 4 and 6.

3 New South Wales has the largest population of gay and other homosexually active men in Australia.

4. The Biomedical Narrative of HIV/AIDS

1 Efficacy 44% but rising to 99% among those who use the drugs daily and are adherent.

2 Efficacy 67% for men, 75% for women.

3 Study stopped as no efficacy shown.

4 Efficacy 62%.

5 No efficacy shown.

6 Efficacy 39%.

7 Condom use, which was initially considered a behavioural prevention strategy, is now deemed by some, for example, Vermund, Tique, Cassell, Pask et al. (2013), to be a biomedical one.

8 As social scientists, we wonder what disciplines inform 'implementation science'.

9 It is interesting to note, however, that those in the United States who were opposed to
   needle and syringe programmes (NSPs, or 'exchanges' as they were called) argued that
   as there had been no RCT to demonstrate the efficacy of NSPs, they should not be
   promoted as a form of HIV prevention.

10 The decline in HIV in this population is not surprising given that people who inject
   drugs are likely to prefer to use sterile needles and syringes when available and, hence,
   there was little likelihood of any risk compensation, which remains a concern in populations where sexual intercourse is the major mode of HIV-transmission and where
   condoms provide the most effective prevention.

5. Risk and Vulnerability

1 The term 'bisexual transmission', used by some to refer to contracting HIV via engaging in sex with a bisexual, illustrates this conflation.

2 Testing pregnant women became more acceptable after 1996 when, with the development of ART, perinatal transmission could be significantly reduced by treating HIV-
   positive pregnant women.

6. Social Practices of Communities

1 Allman discusses the role of community in social and behavioural science research and
   presents an argument about the harms of framing social science, conducted outside of a
   community-engaged framework, as science that has somehow failed (Allman, 2013).

7. Researching Social Change, Working
with Contingency

1 Wilson et al. (2008) report that that the proportion of people on ART with undetectable
   viral load has increased to 90% at 400 copies/ml sensitivity and 85% at 50 copies/ml
   sensitivity.

2 It is of interest to note that serodiscordant heterosexual couples interviewed in Sydney
   in 2009, many of whom engaged in unprotected vaginal intercourse prior to knowing about the Swiss Consensus Statement, were overwhelmingly sceptical of the Swiss
   Consensus Statement's prevention message (Persson, 2010).

3 These figures do not add up to 100% as there was an additional category of HIV-
   prevention research, not discussed here, of 'epidemiological research'.

4 With reference to recent PrEP trials, McMichael & Rosengarten (2013) demonstrate
   that the ways in which RCTs are conducted can and do produce inconsistent results.

5 Cohen et al. (2012) note that although the iPrEx trial reported no increase in sexual
   risk behaviour, the behaviour of individuals in real-world settings may be different. It is
   highly likely that individuals using PrEP will forego condom use.

6 When an anthropologist from Senegal, Cheikh Niang, at the 2012 meeting (in Cape
   Town) of the Global HIV Prevention Working Group (comprised mainly of biomedical scientists) pointed out that male circumcision carries a complex significance, with
   multiple and interconnected dimensions – religious, spiritual, social, biomedical, aes-
   thetic and cultural – and that creating such a 'demand' might also raise questions in

association with female circumcision, there was silence. A year later, at a workshop organised by public health researchers at Johns Hopkins, a medical epidemiologist from the United States who expressed concern about the slow uptake of male circumcision in Botswana, was taken aback when Susan Kippax presented her with the following scenario: How, she was asked, would US citizens be likely to respond to health messages (based on efficacy trials using RCTs) promoting female genital mutilation for the prevention of, for the sake for argument, cervical cancer.

REFERENCES

Abdool Karim, Q., Abdool Karim, S. S., Frolich, J. A., Grobler, A. C., Baxter, C., Mansoor, L. E. ... Taylor, D., on behalf of the CAPRISA 004 Trial Group. (2010). Effectiveness and safety of tenofovir gel, an antiretroviral microbicide, for the prevention of HIV infection in women. *Science, 329*, 1168–1174.

Adam, B. (2005). Constructing the neoliberal sexual actor: Responsibility and care of the self in the discourse of barebackers. *Culture, Health & Sexuality, 7*, 333–346.

———. (2011). Epistemic fault lines in biomedical and social approaches to HIV prevention. *Journal of the International AIDS Society, 14* (Suppl. 2), S2.

Adamchack, S., Kiragu, K., Watson, C., Muhwezi, M., Nelson, T., Akia-Fiedler, A., Kibombo, R. & Juma, M. (2007). *The Straight Talk Campaign in Uganda: Impact of Mass Media Initiatives, Summary Report.* Horizons Final Report. Washington, DC: Population Council.

Aggleton, P. & Kippax, S. (2014). Australia's HIV-prevention Response: Introduction to Special Issue. *AIDS Education & Prevention, 26*, 187–190.

Aggleton, P. & Parker, R. (2015). Moving beyond the biomedicalization of the HIV response: Implications for community involvement and community leadership among MSM and transgender people. *American Journal of Public Health, 105*, 1552–1558.

aids2031 Social Drivers Working Group (2010). *Revolutionizing the AIDS Response: Building AIDS Resilient Communities* (aids2031 Social Drivers Working Group report). Worcester, MA: Clark University and the International Center for Research on Women.

Allen, S., Meinzen-Derr, J., Kautzman, M., Zulu, I., Trask, S., Fideli, U., Musonda, R., Kasolo, F., Gao, F. & Haworth, A. (2003). Sexual behaviour of HIV discordant couples after HIV counseling and testing. *AIDS, 17*, 733–740.

Allen, T. (2006). AIDS and evidence: Interrogating some Ugandan myths. *Journal of Biosocial Science, 38*, 7–28.

Allen, T. & Heald. S. (2004). HIV/AIDS Policy in Africa: What has worked in Uganda and what has failed in Botswana? *Journal of International Development, 16*, 1141–1154.

Allman, D. (2013). Community centrality and social science research. Paper presented at the Second International HIV Social Sciences and Humanities Conference, Paris.

Altman, D. (1994). *Power and Community: Organizational and Cultural Responses to AIDS.* London: Taylor and Francis.

———. (2006). Taboos and denial in government responses. *International Affairs, 82*, 257–268.

———. (2013). *The End of the Homosexual?* Queensland, Australia: University of Queensland Press.

ANCAHRD (2001). *Guidelines for the Management and Post Exposure Prophylaxis of Individuals who Sustain Nonoccupational Exposure to HIV.* Bulletin No. 28, July. Canberra: Australian Government Department of Health.

Anderson, R. (2000). Prevention works. Plenary paper presented at the 13th International AIDS Conference, Durban, South Africa.

Ankrah, E. M. (1992). Aids in Uganda: Initial social work. *Journal of Social Development in Africa, 7*, 53–61.

Aral, S. O. & Peterman, T. A. (1999). Do we know the effectiveness of behavioural interventions? *The Lancet, 351*, 33–36.

Asiimwe-Okiror, G., Opio, A. A., Musinguzi, J., Madraa, E., Tembo, G. & Caraël, M. (1997). Change in sexual behaviour and decline in HIV infection among young pregnant women in urban Uganda. *AIDS, 11*, 1757–1763.

Auerbach, J. D., Parkhurst, J. O. & Cáceres C. F. (2011). Addressing social drivers of HIV/AIDS for the long-term response: Conceptual and methodological considerations. *Global Public Health, 6* (Suppl. 3), S293–S309.

Auvert, B., Taljaard, D., Lagarde, E., Sobngwi-Tambeko, J., Sitta, R. & Puren, A. (2005). Randomised, controlled intervention trial of male circumcision for reduction of HIV infection risk: The ANRS 1265 Trial. *PLoS Medicine, 2*, e298.

Ayres, J. R., Paiva, V. & Franca, I. Jr. (2011). From the natural history of disease to vulnerability: Changing concepts and practices in public health. In *Routledge Handbook of Public Health*, edited by R. Parker & M. Sommer, 98–107. London: Routledge.

Baeten, J. M., Donnell, D., Ndase, P., Mugo, N. R., Campbell, J. D., Wangisi, J. ... Partners PrEP Study Team (2012). Antiretroviral prophylaxis for HIV prevention in heterosexual men and women. *The New England Journal of Medicine, 367*, 399–410.

Bailey, R. C., Moses, S., Parker, C. B., Agot, K., MacLean I., Kieger, J. N. ... Ndinya-Achola, J. O. (2007). Male circumcision for HIV prevention in young men in Kisumu, Kenya: A randomized trial. *The Lancet, 369*, 643–656.

Baral, S. D., Grosso, A., Holland, C. & Papworth, E. (2014). The epidemiology of HIV among men who have sex with men in countries with generalized HIV epidemics. *Current Opinion in HIV and AIDS, 9*, 156–167.

Barnett, T. & Whiteside, A. (2006). *AIDS in the Twenty-First Century: Disease and Globalization.* 2nd Edition. Palgrave Macmillan: London.

Bass, E. (2005). The two sides of PEPFAR in Uganda. *The Lancet, 365*, 2077–2078.

Bates, J. & Berg, R. (2014). Sex workers as safe sex advocates: Sex workers protect both themselves and the wider community from HIV. *AIDS Education & Prevention, 26*, 191–201.

Baum, F. (2008). *The New Public Health.* South Melbourne: Oxford University Press.

Bavington, B. (2013). The Opposites Attract Study: HIV treatment as prevention among gay male sero-discordant relationships. Paper presented at Kirby Institute Inaugural Symposium, UNSW, Sydney, Australia.

Bekker, L-G. & Hosek, S. (2015). Building our youth for the future. *Journal of the International AIDS Society, 18* (Suppl. 1), 20027.

Bell, S. A. (2011). Young people and sexual agency in rural Uganda. *Culture, Health & Sexuality, 14*, 283–296.

Bell, S. A. & Aggleton, P. (2012). Time to invest in a 'counterpublic health' approach: Promoting sexual health amongst sexually active young people in rural Uganda. *Children's Geographies, 10*, 385–397.

Berkman, A., Garcia, J., Munoz-Laboy, M., Paiva, V. & Parker, R. (2005). A critical analysis of the Brazilian response to HIV/AIDS: Lessons learned for controlling and mitigating the epidemic in developing countries. *American Journal of Public Health, 95*, 1162–1172.

Bernard, D., Kippax, S. & Baxter, D. (2008). Effective partnership and adequate investment underpin a successful response: Key factors in dealing with HIV increases. *Sexual Health, 5*, 193–201.

Botswana National AIDS Coordinating Agency (2014). *Global AIDS Response Report: Progress Report of the National Response to the 2011 Declaration of Commitments on HIV & AIDS.* Gaborone: Botswana National AIDS Coordinating Agency.

Bourdieu, P. (1986). The forms of capital. In *Handbook of Theory and Research for the Sociology of Education*, edited by J. Richardson, 46–58. Westport, CT: Greenwood Press.

———. (1998). *Practical Reason: On the Theory of Action.* Stanford, CA: Stanford University Press.

Bourgois, P. & Scheper-Hughes, N. (2004). Commentary on Farmer, P. (2004), An anthropology of structural violence. *Current Anthropology, 45*, 317–318.

Bowtell, W. (2005). *Australia's Response to HIV/AIDS 1982–2005.* Report prepared for Research and Dialogue Project on Regional Responses to the Spread of HIV/AIDS in East Asia Organised by the Japan Center for International Exchange and the Friends of the Global Fund to Fight AIDS Tuberculosis and Malaria (Japan). Sydney: Lowy Institute for International Policy.

Brown, G., O'Donnell, D., Crooks, L. & Lake, R. (2014). Mobilisation, politics, investment and constant adaptation: Lessons from the Australian health promotion response to HIV. *Health Promotion Journal of Australia, 25*, 35–41.

Burke, M., Rajabu, M. & Kippax, S. (2004). Foundational issues in VCT in a PMTCT setting in Tanzania. Paper presented at the 16th Annual Conference of the Australasian Society for HIV Medicine, Canberra, Australia.

Burns, K. (2009). *Human Rights, Gender and Mandatory Testing.* New York: Law and Health Initiative, Open Society Institute.

Buve, A., Bishikwabo-Nsarhaza, K. & Mutangadura, G. (2002). The spread and effect of HIV-infection in sub-Saharan Africa. *The Lancet, 359*, 2011–2017.

Caceres, C. & Race, K. (2010). Knowledge, power and HIV/AIDS: Research and the global response. In *Routledge Handbook of Sexuality, Health and Rights*, edited by P. Aggleton & R. Parker, 175–183. London and New York: Routledge.

Camargo, de, K. R. (2009). Celebrating the 20th anniversary of Ulysses Guimarães' rebirth of Brazilian democracy and the creation of Brazil's national health care system. *American Journal of Public Health, 99*, 30–31.

Campbell C. A. (2003). *Letting Them Die: How HIV/AIDS Prevention Programmes Often Fail.* Bloomington, IN: Indiana University Press.

———. (2009). Building AIDS competent communities: Possibilities and challenges. Paper presented at Mobilizing Social Capital in a World with AIDS, Salzburg, Austria.

———. (2010). Technologies of 'participation' and 'capacity building' in HIV/AIDS management in Africa: Four case studies. In *HIV Treatment and Prevention Technologies in International Perspective*, edited by M. Davis & C. Squire, 18–32. Basingstoke: Palgrave Macmillan.

Campbell, C. A., Nair, Y. & Maimane, S. (2007). Building contexts that support effective community responses to HIV/AIDS: A South African case study. *American Journal of Community Psychology, 39*, 347–363.

Cardo, D. M., Culver, D. H., Ciesielski, C. A., Srivastata, P. U., Marcus, R., Abiteboul, D., Heppenstall, J., Ippolito, G., Lot, F., McKibben, P. S. & Bell, D. M. (1997). A case-control study of HIV seroconversion in health care workers after percutaneous exposure. *New England Journal of Medicine, 337*, 1485–1490.

Carey, R. F., Herman, W. A., Retta, S. M., Rinaldi, J. E., Herman, B. A. & Athey, T. W. (1992). Effectiveness of latex condoms as a barrier to Human Immunodeficiency Virus-sized particles under conditions of simulated use. *Sexually Transmitted Diseases, 19*, 230–234.

Castells, M. (1997). *The Power of Identity*. Malden, MN: Blackwell.

CDC (2003). Advancing HIV Prevention: New Strategies for a Changing Epidemic – United States, MMWR: *Morbidity and Mortality Weekly Report, 52,* 329–332.

CDC e-Hap FYI Updates (2014). *New Guidelines Recommend Daily HIV Prevention Pill for Those at Substantial Risk*. Retrieved from http://content.govdelivery.com/accounts/USCDC/bulletins/b7c7a2

Chan, B. T., Weiser, S. D., Boum, Y. Siedner, M. J., Mocello, A. R., Haberer, J. E. ... Tsai, A. C. (2015). Persistent HIV-related stigma in rural Uganda during a period of increasing HIV incidence despite treatment expansion. *AIDS, 29,* 83–90.

Chen, L., Jha, P., Stirling, B., Sgaier, S., Daid, T., Kaul, R., Nagelkerke, N. for the International Studies of HIV/AIDS (ISHA) Investigators. (2007). Sexual risk factors for HIV infection in early and advanced HIV epidemics in sub-Saharan Africa: Systematic overview of 68 epidemiological studies. *PLoS One, 2,* e1001.

Clark, D. B. (1973). The concept of community: A re-examination. *The Sociological Review, 21,* 397–416.

Clatts, M. C. (1994). All the king's horses and all the king's men: Some personal reflections on ten years of AIDS ethnography. *Human Organization, 53,* 93–95.

Cleland, J. & Watkins, S. (2006). Sex without birth or death: A comparison of two international humanitarian movements. In *Social Information Transmission and Human Biology*, edited by J. Wells, S. Strickland & K. Laland, 207–223. Boca Raton, FL: Taylor & Francis.

Clinton, H. R. (2011, December). Remarks on 'Creating an AIDS-Free Generation'. Speech given to National Institutes of Health, Masur Auditorium, Bethesda, MD. Retrieved from http://www.state.gov/secretary/rm/2011/11/1768.10.htm.

Coates, T. J., Richter, L. & Caceres, C. (2008). Behavioural strategies to reduce HIV transmission: How to make them work better. *The Lancet, 372,* 669–684.

Cohen, Jon (2011). HIV treatment as prevention. *Science, 334,* 1628.

Cohen, Jonathan, Schleifer, R. & Tate, T. (2005). AIDS in Uganda: The human-rights dimension. *The Lancet, 365,* 2075–2076.

Cohen, Jonathan & Tate, T. (2006). The less they know, the better: Abstinence-only HIV/AIDS Programs in Uganda. *Reproductive Health Matters, 14,* 174–178.

Cohen, M. S., Chen, Y. Q., McCauley, M., Gamble, T., Hosseinipour, M. C., Kumarasamy, N. ... HPTN 052 Study Team (2011). Prevention of HIV-1 infection with early antiretroviral therapy. *New England Journal of Medicine, 365,* 493–505.

Cohen, M. S., Muessig, K. E., Kumi Smith, M., Powers, K. A. & Kashuba, A. D. M. (2012). Antiviral agents and HIV prevention: Controversies, conflicts and consensus. Editorial Review, *AIDS, 26,* 1585–1598.

Cohen, M. S., McCauley, M. & Gamble, T. (2012). HIV treatment as prevention and HPTN052. Review, *Current Opinion in HIV and AIDS, 7,* 99–105.

Cooper, M. (2015). The Theology of Emergency – Welfare Reform, US Foreign Aid, and the Faith-based Initiative. *Theory, Culture & Society, 32,* 53–77.

Cosgrave, J., Fairchild, A. & Rosner, D. (2013). The history of structural approaches in public health. In *Structural Approaches in Public Health*, edited by M. Sommer & R. Parker, 17–27. London: Routledge.

Crawford, J., Rodden, P., Kippax, S. & Van de Ven, P. (2001). Negotiated safety and other agreements between men in relationships: Risk practice redefined. *International Journal of STD & AIDS, 12,* 164–170.

Daniel, H. & Parker, R. (1993). *Sexuality, Politics and AIDS in Brazil*. London: The Falmer Press.

Das, M., Chu, P. L. Santos, G. M., Scheer, S., Vintinghoff, E., McFarland, W. & Colfax, G. (2010). Decreases in community viral load are accompanied by reductions in new HIV infections in San Francisco. *PLoS One, 5*, e11068.

Davidovich, U., de Wit, J. & Stroebe, W. (2000). Assessing sexual risk behaviour of young gay men in primary relationships: The incorporation of negotiated safety and negotiated safety compliance. *AIDS, 14*, 701–706.

Denison, J. A., O'Reilly, K. R., Schmid, G. P., Kennedy, C. E. & Sweat, M. D. (2008). HIV voluntary counselling and testing and behavioral risk reduction in developing countries: A meta-analysis, 1990–2005. *AIDS and Behavior, 12*, 363–373.

Denning, P., Nakashima, A. K. & Wortley, P. (2000). Increasing rates of unprotected anal intercourse among HIV-infected men who have sex with men in the United States. Paper presented at the 13th International AIDS Conference, Durban, South Africa.

Des Jarlais, D. C., Hagan, H., Friedman, S. R., Friedmann, P., Goldberg, D., Frischer, M. … Myers, T. (1995). Maintaining low HIV seroprevalence in populations of injecting drug users. *Journal of the American Medical Association, 274*, 1226–1231.

Dodds, J. P., Nardone, A., Mercey, D. E. & Johnson, A. M. (2000). Increase in high risk sexual behaviour among homosexual men, London 1996–8: Cross sectional, questionnaire study. *British Medical Journal, 320*, 1510–1511.

Drucker, E. (2012). Failed drug policies in the United States and the future of AIDS: A perfect storm. *Journal of Public Health Policy, 33*, 309–316.

Dubois-Arber, F., Masur, J.-B., Hausser, D., Zimmerman, E. & Paccaud, F. (1993). Evaluation of AIDS prevention among homosexual and bisexual men in Switzerland. *Social Science & Medicine, 37*, 1539–1544.

Dubois-Arber, F., Jeannin, A. & Spencer, B. (1999). Long term global evaluation of a national AIDS prevention strategy: The case of Switzerland. *AIDS, 13*, 2571–2582.

Dubois-Arber, F., Jeannin, A., Meystre-Agustoni, G., Spencer, B., Moreau-Gruet, F., Balthasar, H., Benninghoff, F., Klaue, K. & Paccauld, F. (2003). *Evaluation of the HIV/AIDS Prevention Strategy in Switzerland: Abridged Version of Seventh Synthesis Report 1999–2003.* Lausanne: Institut Universitaire de Medecine de Sociale et Preventive.

Dukers, N., de Wit, J., Goudsmit, J., Couthino, R. (2000). Recent increase in sexual risk behavior and sexually transmitted diseases in a cohort of homosexual men: The price of highly active anti-retroviral therapy? Paper presented at the 13th International AIDS Conference, Durban, South Africa.

Dworkin, S. & Blankenship, K. (2009). Microfinance and HIV/AIDS prevention: Assessing its promise and limitations. *AIDS and Behavior, 13*, 463–469.

Ekstrand, M. L., Stall, R. D., Paul, J. P., Osmond, D. H. & Coates, T. J. (2000). Gay men report high rates of unprotected sex with partners of unknown or discordant HIV status. *AIDS, 13*, 1525–1533.

Epstein, H. (2007). *The Invisible Cure.* New York: Picador.

Fairley, C., Grulich, A., Imrie, J. & Pitts, M. (2008). Introductory Editorial: The analysis of a natural experiment in HIV control. *Sexual Health, 5*, 89.

Fallon, S. J. & Forrest, D. W. (2012). Unexamined challenges to applying the treatment as prevention model among men who have sex with men in the United States: A community public health perspective. *AIDS and Behavior, 16*, 1739–1742.

Farmer, P. (1992). *AIDS and Accusation: Haiti and the Geography of Blame.* Berkeley: University of California Press.

———. (2004). An anthropology of structural violence. *Current Anthropology, 45*, 305–317.

Farmer, P., Connors, M. & Simmons, J. (1996). *Women, Poverty and AIDS: Sex, Drugs and Structural Violence.* Monroe, ME: Common Courage Press.

Fassin, D. (2007). *When Bodies Remember: Experiences and Politics of AIDS in South Africa*. Berkeley and Los Angeles: University of California Press.

Friedman, S. R. & Reid, G. (2002). The need for dialectical models as shown in the response to the HIV/AIDS epidemic. *International Journal of Social Science Policy, 22*, 177–200.

Friedman, S.R., Kippax, S., Phaswana-Mafuya, N., Rossi, D. & Newman, C. (2006). Emerging future issues in HIV/AIDS social research, *AIDS, 20*, 959–965.

Friedman, S.R., de Jong, W., Rossi, D., Touze, G., Rockwell, R., Des Jarlais, D. C. & Elovich, R. (2007a). Harm reduction theory: Users' culture, micro-social indigenous harm reduction, and the self-organization and outside-organizing of users' groups. *International Journal of Drug Policy, 18*, 107–117.

Friedman, S.R., Mateu-Gelabert, P., Curtis, R., Maslow, C., Bolyard, M., Sandoval, M. & Flom, P. L. (2007b). Social capital or networks, negotiations and norms? A neighbourhood case study. *American Journal of Preventive Medicine, 32* (Suppl. 6), S160–S170.

Fumento, M. (1990). *The Myth of Heterosexual AIDS: How a Tragedy Has Been Distorted by the Media and Partisan Politics*. New York: Basic Books.

Fylkesnes, K., Haworth, A., Rosensvard, C. & Mushimwa Kwapa, P. (1999). HIV counseling and testing: Overemphasizing high acceptance rates a threat to confidentiality and the right not to know, *AIDS, 13*, 2469–2474.

Gale, M., Holden, J., Selvey, C., Chant, K. & Whittaker, B. (2014). Eliminating HIV transmission in New South Wales: The critical role of testing. *Medical Journal of Australia, 201*, 260–262.

Garnett, G. P., Becker, S. & Bertozzi, S. (2012). Treatment as prevention: Translating efficacy trials to population effectiveness. *Current Opinion in HIV and AIDS, 7*, 157–163.

Gibbs, A., Willan, S., Misselhorn, A. & Mangoma, J. (2012). Combined structural interventions for gender equality and livelihood security: A critical review of the evidence from southern and eastern Africa and the implications for young people. *Journal of the International AIDS Society, 15* (Suppl. 1), 17362.

Gisselquist, D., Potterat, J. J. & Brody, S. (2004). Running on empty: Sexual cofactors are insufficient to drive Africa's turbocharged HIV epidemic. *International Journal of STD and AIDS, 15*, 442–452.

Global HIV Prevention Working Group (2002). *Global Mobilization for HIV Prevention: A Blueprint for Action*. Retrieved from http://www.issuelab.org/resource/global_mobilization_for_hiv_prevention_a_blueprint_for_action

———. (2003). *Access to HIV Prevention: Closing the Gap*. Retrieved from http://www.issuelab.org/resource/access_to_hiv_prevention_closing_the_gap

———. (2004). *HIV Prevention in the Era of Expanded Treatment Access*. Retrieved from http://www.unicef.org/aids/files/HIV-Prevention-in-the-Era-of-Expanded-Treatment-Access.pdf

———. (2006). *New Approaches to HIV Prevention: Accelerating Research and Ensuring Future Access*. Retrieved from http://www.issuelab.org/resource/new_approaches_to_hiv_prevention_accelerating_research_and_ensuring_future_access

———. (2007). *Bringing HIV Prevention to Scale: An Urgent Global Priority*. Retrieved from http://www.iasociety.org/web/webcontent/file/pwg-hiv_prevention_report_final.pdf

———. (2008). *Behavior Change and HIV Prevention: [Re]Considerations for the 21st Century*. Retrieved from http://kaiserfamilyfoundation.files.wordpress.com/2013/01/pwg080508fullreport.pdf

GNP+, UNAIDS (2011). *Positive Health, Dignity and Prevention: A Policy Framework*. Amsterdam: GNP+. Retrieved from http://www.unaids.org/sites/default/files/media_asset/20110701_PHDP_0.pdf

Granich, R. M., Gilks, C. F., Dye, C., de Cock, K. M. & Williams, B. G. (2009). Universal voluntary HIV testing with immediate antiretroviral therapy as a strategy for the elimination of HIV transmission: A mathematical model. *The Lancet, 373*, 48–57.

Granich, R., Crowley, S., Vitoria, M., Smyth, C., Kahn, J. G., Bennett, R., Ying-Ru, L., Souteyrand, Y. & Williams, B. (2010). Highly active antiretroviral treatment as prevention of HIV transmission: A review of scientific evidence and uptake. *Current Opinion in HIV and AIDS, 5*, 298–304.

Granich, R., Williams, B. & Montaner, J. (2013). Fifteen million people on antiretroviral treatment by 2015: Treatment as prevention. *Current Opinion in HIV and AIDS, 8*, 41–49.

Grant, R. M., Lama, J. R., Anderson, P. L., McMahan, V., Liu, A. Y., Vargas, L. ... iPrEx Study Team. (2010). Preexposure chemopdophlaxis for HIV prevention in men who have sex with men. *New England Journal of Medicine, 363*, 2587–2599.

Grassly, N. C., Lowndes, C. M., Rhodes, T., Judd, A., Renton, A. & Garnett, G. P. (2003). Modelling emerging HIV epidemics: The role of injecting drug use and sexual transmission in the Russian Federation, China and India. *International Journal of Drug Policy, 14*, 25–43.

Gray, R. H., Serwadda, D., Kigozi, G., Nalugoda, F. & Wawer, M. J. (2006). Uganda's HIV prevention success: The role of sexual behavior change and the national response. Commentary on Green et al. (2006). *AIDS and Behavior, 10*, 347–350.

Gray, R. H., Kigozi, G., Serwadda, D., Makumbi, F., Watya, S., Nalugoda, F. ... Wawer, M. J. (2007). Male circumcision for HIV prevention in men in Rakai, Uganda: A randomised trial. *The Lancet, 369*, 657–666.

Gray, R. H., Kigozi, G., Kong, X., Ssempiija, V., Makumbi, F., Wattya, S. ... Wawer, M. J. (2012). The effectiveness of male circumcision for HIV prevention and effects on risk behaviors in a posttrial follow-up study. *AIDS, 26*, 609–615.

Green, A. & Kolar, K. (2014). Engineering behaviour change in an epidemic: The epistemology of NIH-funded HIV prevention science. *Sociology of Health & Illness, 37*, 561–577.

Green, E. C. Halperin, D. T., Nantulya, V. & Hogle, J. (2006). Uganda's HIV Prevention Success: The Role of Sexual Behavior Change and the National Response. *AIDS and Behavior, 10*, 335–346.

Green, E. C. & Ruark, A. (2011). *AIDS, Behaviour and Culture: Understanding Evidence-based Prevention*. Walnut Creek, CA: Left Coast Press.

Green, E. C., Kajubi, P., Ruark, A., Kamya, S., D'Errico, N. & Hearst, N. (2013). The need to reemphasize behavior change for HIV prevention in Uganda: A qualitative study. *Studies in Family Planning, 44*, 25–43.

Gregson, S, Garnett, G. P., Nyamukupa, C. A., Hallett, T. B., Lewis, J. J., Mason, P. R., Chandiwana, S. K. & Anderson, R. M. (2006). HIV decline associated with behaviour change in eastern Zimbabwe. *Science, 311*, 664–666.

Grinstead, O. A., Gregorich, S. E., Choi, K-H., Coates, T. & the Voluntary HIV-1 Counselling and Testing Efficacy Study Group (2001). Positive and negative life events after counselling and testing: the Voluntary HIV-1 Counselling and Testing Efficacy Study. *AIDS, 15*, 1045–1052.

Grunseit, A. & Kippax, S. (1993). *Effects of Sex Education on Young People's Sexual Behaviour*, Geneva; WHO/GPA (updated and published by UNAIDS, 1997). Retrieved from http://data.unaids.org/publications/IRC-pub01/jc010-impactyoungpeople_en.pdf.

Hallett, T. B., Aberle-Grasse, J., Bello, G., Boulos, L. M., Cayemittes, M. P., Cheluget, B. ... Walker, N. (2006). Declines in HIV prevalence can be associated with changing sexual behaviour in Uganda, urban Kenya, Zimbabwe, and urban Haiti. *Sexually Transmissible Infections, 82* (Suppl. 1), 1–8.

Halperin, D. T., Mugurungi, O., Hallett, T. B., Muchini, B., Campbell, B., Magure, T., Benedikt, C. & Gregson, S. (2011). A surprising prevention success: Why did the HIV epidemic decline in Zimbabwe? *PLoS Medicine, 8*, e1000414.

Hanenberg, R. S., Rojanapithayakorn, W., Kunasol, P. & Sokal, D. C. (1994). Impact of Thailand's HIV-control programme as indicated by the decline in sexually transmitted diseases. *The Lancet, 344*, 243–245.

Hargreaves, J. R., Slaymaker, E., Fearon, E. & Howe, L. D. (2012). Changes over time in sexual behaviour among young people with different levels of educational attainment in Tanzania. *Journal of the International AIDS Society, 15* (Suppl. 1), 17363.

Harré, R. (1979). *Social Being.* Oxford: Basil Blackwell.

Henderson, K., Worth, H., Aggleton, P. & Kippax, S. (2009). Enhancing HIV prevention: Renewing the social and behavioural agenda. *Global Public Health, 4*, 117–130.

Holmes, W. (2005). Seeking rational policy settings for PMTCT, *The Lancet, 366*, 1835–1836.

Holt, M. (2011). Gay men and ambivalence about 'gay community': From gay community attachment to personal communities. *Culture Health & Sexuality, 13*, 857–871.

———. (2014). Gay men's HIV risk reduction practices: the influence of epistemic communities in HIV social and behavioural research. *AIDS Education & Prevention, 26*, 214–223.

Holt, M., Murphy, D. A., Callander, D., Ellard, J., Rosengarten, M., Kippax, S. C. & de Wit, J. (2012). Willingness to use HIV pre-exposure prophylaxis and the likelihood of decreased condom use are both associated with unprotected anal intercourse and the perceived likelihood of becoming HIV positive among Australian gay and bisexual men. *Sexually Transmitted Infections, 88*, 258–263.

Holt, M., Lea, T., Murphy, D., Ellard, J., Rosengarten, M., Kippax, S. & de Wit, J. (2014a). Willingness to use HIV pre-exposure prophylaxis has declined among Australian gay and bisexual men: Results from repeated, cross-sectional surveys, 2011–2013. *Journal of Acquired Immune Deficiency Syndromes, 67*, 222–226.

Holt, M., Lea, T., Murphy, D., Ellard, J., Rosengarten, M., Kippax, S. & de Wit, J. (2014b). Australian gay and bisexual men's attitudes to HIV treatment as prevention in repeated, national surveys, 2011–2013. *PLOS ONE, 9*, e112349.

Holtgrave, D. R., Maulsby, C., Wehrmeyer, L. & Hall, H. I. (2012). Behavioural factors in assessing impact of HIV treatment as prevention. *AIDS and Behavior, 16*, 1085–1091.

Human Rights Watch (2005). *The Less They Know, the Better: Abstinence-Only HIV/AIDS Programs in Uganda, 17*, 4(A). Authored by Cohen, J. & Tate, T. Retrieved from http://www.hrw.org/reports/2005/03/29/less-they-know-better-0

Iyer, P. & Aggleton, P. (2014). 'Virginity is a virtue: Prevent early sex' – Teacher perceptions of sex education in a Ugandan secondary school. *British Journal of Sociology of Education, 35*, 432–448.

Jewkes, R., Nduna, M., Levin, J., Jama, N., Dunkle, K. & Puren, A. (2008). Impact of Stepping Stones on incidence of HIV and HSV-2 and sexual behaviour in rural South Africa: cluster randomised controlled trial. *British Medical Journal, 337*, 391–395.

Jia, Z., Ruan, Y., Li, Q., Xie, P., Li, P., Wang, X., Chen, R.Y. & Shao, Y. (2013). Antiretroviral therapy to prevent HIV transmission in serodiscordant couples in China (2003–11): A national observational cohort study. *The Lancet, 382*, 1195–1203.

Jin, F., Crawford, J., Prestage, G., Zablotska, I., Imrie, J., Kippax, S., Kaldor, J. & Grulich, A. (2009). Unprotected anal intercourse, risk reduction behaviours, and subsequent HIV infection in a cohort of homosexual men. *AIDS, 23*, 243–252.

Jin, F., Jansson, J., Law, M., Prestage, G., Zablotska, I., Imrie, J., Kippax, S., Kaldor, J., Grulich, A. & Wilson, D. (2010). Per-contact probability of HIV transmission in homosexual men in Sydney in the era of HAART. *AIDS*, *24*, 907–910.

Jones, T. & Mitchell, A. (2014). Young people in HIV prevention in Australian schools. *AIDS Education & Prevention*, *26*, 224–233.

Kalichman, S. C. & Simbayi, L. C. (2003). HIV Testing attitudes, AIDS stigma, and voluntary counselling and testing in a black township in Cape Town, South Africa, *Sexually Transmitted Infections*, *79*, 442–447.

Kinder, P. (1996). A new prevention education strategy for gay men: Responding to the impact of AIDS on gay men's lives. Paper presented at 11th International AIDS Conference, Vancouver, Canada.

Kippax, S. (2003). Sexual health interventions are unsuitable for experimental evaluation. In *Effective Sexual Health Interventions: Issues in Experimental Evaluation*, edited by J. M. Stephenson, J. Imrie & C. Bonell, 17–34. Oxford: Oxford University Press.

———. (2006). A public health dilemma: A testing question. *AIDS Care*, *18*, 230–235.

———. (2008). Understanding and integrating the structural and biomedical determinants of HIV-infection: A way forward for prevention. *Current Opinion in HIV and AIDS*, *3*, 489–494.

———. (2012). Effective HIV prevention: the indispensable role of social science. *Journal of the International AIDS Society*, *15*, 17357.

Kippax, S., Crawford, J., Davis, M., Rodden, P. & Dowsett, G. W. (1993). Sustaining safe sex: A longitudinal study of a sample of homosexual men, *AIDS*, *7*, 257–263.

Kippax, S. & Crawford, J. (1995). Prophylactic vaccine trials: What is different about HIV? *Venereology*, *8*, 178–182.

Kippax, S., Noble, J., Prestage, G., Crawford, J. M., Campbell, D., Baxter, D. & Cooper, D. (1997). Sexual negotiation in the 'AIDS era': Negotiated safety revisited, *AIDS*, *11*, 191–197.

Kippax, S. & Kinder, P. (2002). Reflexive practice: The relationship between social research and health promotion in HIV prevention, *Sex Education*, *2*, 91–104.

Kippax, S. & Race, K. (2003). Sustaining safe practice: Twenty years on. *Social Science & Medicine*, *57*, 1–12.

Kippax, S. & Stephenson, N. (2005). Meaningful evaluation of sex and relationship education. *Sex Education*, *5*, 359–373.

Kippax, S. & Stephenson, N. (2012). Beyond the distinction between biomedical and social dimensions of HIV: Prevention through the lens of a social public health. *American Journal of Public Health*, *102*, 789–799.

Kippax, S., Stephenson, N., Parker, R. & Aggleton, P. (2013). Between agency and structure in HIV prevention: Understanding the middle ground of social practice. *American Journal of Public Health*, *103*, 1367–1375.

The Kirby Institute (2009). *HIV, Viral Hepatitis and Sexually Transmissible Infections in Australia: Annual Surveillance Report, 2009*. The Kirby Institute, University of New South Wales.

———. (2014). *HIV, Viral Hepatitis and Sexually Transmissible Infections in Australia: Annual Surveillance Report, 2014*. The Kirby Institute, University of New South Wales.

Krieger, N. (2008). Proximal, distal, and the politics of causation: What has level got to do with it? *American Journal of Public Health*, *98*, 221–230.

Kretzschmar, M., Schim van der Loeff, M. & Coutinho, R. (2012). Elimination of HIV by test and treat: A phantom of wishful thinking! *AIDS*, *26*, 247–251.

Lallemant, M., Jourdain, G., Le Coeur, S., Mary J. Y., Ngo-Giang-Huong, N., Koetsawang, S. ... Thaineua, V. (2004). Single-dose perinatal nevirapine plus standard zidovudine to prevent mother-to-child transmission of HIV-1 in Thailand. *New England Journal of Medicine*, *351*, 217–228.

Lancet Editorial (2011). HIV treatment as prevention – it works. *The Lancet*, *377*, 1719.

Lancet Infectious Diseases Editorial (2011). Treatment as prevention for HIV. *The Lancet Infectious Diseases*, *11*, 651.

Lawless, S., Kippax, S. & Crawford, J. (1996). Dirty, diseased and undeserving: The positioning of HIV positive women. *Social Science & Medicine*, *43*, 1371–1377.

Leigh, F. J., Hallett, T. B., Rehle, T. M. & Dorrington, R. E. (2012). The effect of changes in condom usage and antiretroviral treatment coverage on human immunodeficiency virus incidence in South Africa: A model-based analysis. *Journal of the Royal Society Interface*, *9*, 1544–1554.

Leroy, V., Karon, V. M., Alioum, A., Ekpini, E. R., Meda, N., Greenberg, A. E. ... for the West Africa PMTCT Study Group (2002). Twenty-four month efficacy of a maternal short-course zidovudine regimen to prevent mother-to-child transmission of HIV-1 in West Africa. *AIDS*, *16*, 631–641.

Li, X., Lu, H., Ma, X., Sun, Y., He, X., Li, C., ... Jia, Y. (2012). HIV/AIDS-related stigmatizing and discriminatory attitudes and recent HIV testing among men who have sex with men in Beijing. *AIDS and Behavior*, *16*, 499–507.

Lifton, R. J. (1954). Home by ship: Reaction patterns of American prisoners of war repatriated from North Korea. *American Journal of Psychiatry*, *CX*, 732–739.

Low-Beer, D. & Stoneburner, R. (2003). Behaviour and communication change in reducing HIV: Is Uganda unique? *African Journal of AIDS Research*, *2*, 9–12.

Low-Beer, D. & Stoneburner, R. (2004). Uganda and the challenge of HIV/AIDS. In *The Political Economy of AIDS in Africa*, edited by N. Poku & A. Whiteside, 165–190. Aldershot: Ashgate.

Macpherson, E. E., Sadalaki, J., Njoloma, M., Nyongopa, V., Nkhwazi, L., Mwapasa, V. ... Theobold, S. (2012). Transactional sex and HIV: Understanding the gendered structural drivers of HIV in fishing communities in Southern Malawi. *Journal of the International AIDS Society*, *15* (Suppl. 1), 17364.

Madden, A. & Wodak, A. (2014). Australia's response to HIV among people who inject drugs. *AIDS Education & Prevention*, *26*, 234–244.

Maggiolo, F. & Leone, S. (2010). Is HAART modifying the HIV epidemic? *The Lancet*, *376*, 492–493.

Malaysian Ministry of Health (2014). *Malaysia 2014, Country Response to HIV/AIDS*. Putrajaya: HIV/STI Section, Disease Control Division, Malaysian Ministry of Health.

Maman, S., Mbwambo, J., Hogan, N. M., Kilonzo, G. P. & Sweat, M. (2001). Women's barriers to HIV-1 testing and disclosure: Challenges for HIV-1 voluntary counseling and testing, *AIDS Care*, *13*, 595–603.

Mann, J., Tarantola, D. & Netter, T. W. (Eds.) (1992). *AIDS in the World: A Global Report*. Cambridge, MA: Harvard University Press.

Marais, H. (2005). *Buckling: The Impact of AIDS in South Africa*. Pretoria: Centre for the Study of AIDS, University of Pretoria.

Marks, G., Crepaz, N. & Janssen, R. S. (2006). Estimating sexual transmission of HIV from persons aware and unaware that they are infected with the virus in the USA. *AIDS*, *20*, 1447–1450.

Mbonye, M., Nalukenge, W., Nakamanya, S., Nalusiba, B., King, R., Vandepitte, J. & Seeley, J. (2012). Gender inequity in the lives of women involved in sex work in Kampala, Uganda. *Journal of the International AIDS Society*, *15* (Suppl. 1), 17365.

Mburu, R. W., Folayan, M. O. & Akanni, O. (2014). The Abuja +12 Declaration: Implications for HIV response in Africa. *African Journal of Reproductive Health*, Special Edition, *18*, 34–46.

McAdam, D., McCarthy, J. D. & Zaid, M. N. (Eds.) (1996). *Comparative Perspectives on Social Movements: Political Opportunities, Mobilizing Structures, and Political Framings*. New York: Cambridge University Press.

McMahon, J. M., Myers, J. E., Kurth, A. E., Cohen, S. E., Mannheimer, S. B., Simmons, J., Pouget, E. R., Trabold, N. & Heberer, J. E. (2014). Oral pre-exposure prophylaxis (PrEP) for prevention of HIV in serodiscordant heterosexual couples in the United States: Opportunities and challenges. *AIDS Patient Care and STDs*, *28*, 462–474.

McMichael, M. & Rosengarten, M. (2013). *Innovation and Biomedicine: Ethics, Evidence and Expectation in HIV.* New York: Palgrave Macmillan.

Mei, S., Quax, R., Van de Vijver, D., Zhu, Y. & Sloot, P. (2011). Increasing risk behaviour can outweigh the benefits of antiretroviral drug treatment on the HIV incidence among men-having-sex-with-men in Amsterdam. *BMC Infectious Diseases*, *11*, 118.

Meinert, L. & Reynolds, S. (2014). Epidemic projectification: AIDS responses in Uganda as event and process. *Cambridge Anthropology*, *32*, 77–94.

Mindel, A. & Kippax, S. (2013). A national strategic approach to improving the health of gay and bisexual men: Experience in Australia. In *The New Public Health and STD/HIV Prevention: Personal, Public and Health System Approaches*, edited by S. O. Aral, K. A. Fenton & J. A. Lipshutz, 339–360. New York: Springer.

Minnis, A. M. & Padian, N. S. (2005). Effectiveness of female controlled barrier methods in preventing sexually transmitted infections and HIV: Current evidence and future research directions. *Sexually Transmitted Infections*, *81*, 193–200.

Montaner, J. S. G. (2013, July 26). *IAS 2013: Julio Montaner* [Video File]. Retrieved from https://www.youtube.com/watch?v=q5-EGcTtyGM

Montaner, J. S. G., Lima, V. D., Barios, R., Yip, B., Wood, E., Kerr, T., Shannon, K., Harrigan, P. R., Hogg, R. S., Daly, P. & Kendall, P. (2010). Association of highly active antiretroviral therapy coverage, population viral load, and yearly new diagnoses in British Columbia, Canada: A population-based study. *The Lancet*, *376*, 532–539.

Muessig, K. E. & Cohen, M. S. (2014). Advances in HIV prevention for serodiscordant couples. *Current HIV/AIDS Report*, *11*, 434–446 .

Murphy, D., Lea, T., de Wit, J., Ellard, J., Kippax, S., Rosengarten, M. & Holt, M. (2015). Interest in using rectal microbicides is associated with perceived HIV vulnerability and engaging in condomless sex with casual partners: Results from a national survey of Australian gay men. *Sexually Transmitted Infections*, *91*, 266–268.

Murray, L. R., Garcia, J., Muñoz-Laboy, M. & Parker, R. (2011). Strange bedfellows: The Catholic Church and Brazilian National AIDS program in the response to AIDS in Brazil. *Social Science & Medicine*, *72*, 945–952.

Neocleous, M. (2013). Resisting resilience. *Radical Philosophy*, *178*, 62.

Nguyen, V-K., Bajos, N., Dubois-Arber, F., O'Malley, J. & Pirkle, C. (2011). Remedicalizing an epidemic: From HIV treatment as prevention to HIV treatment is prevention. *AIDS*, *25*, 291–293.

Niang, C. I. & Boiro, H. (2007). Roundtable: 'You can also cut my finger!': Social construction of male circumcision in West Africa, a case study of Senegal and Guinea-Bissau. *Reproductive Health Matters*, *15*, 22–32.

NSW Health Department (2007). *Consensus Statement. A Think Tank: Why are HIV notifications flat in NSW 1998–2006?* Sydney: NSW Health. Retrieved from http://www.health.nsw. gov.au/sexualhealth/Documents/HIV-consensus-statement.pdf

NSW Ministry of Health (2012). NSW HIV Strategy 2012–2015: A New Era. Sydney: NSW Health. Retrieved from http://www.health.nsw.gov.au/publications/Publications/ nsw-hiv-strategy-2012–15.pdf

Nunn, A. (2009). *The Politics and History of AIDS Treatment in Brazil.* New York: Springer.

Ogden, J., Rao Gupta, G., Williams, W. F. & Warner, A. (2011). Looking back, moving forward: Towards a game-changing response to AIDS. *Global Public Health, 6* (Suppl. 3), S285–S292.

Padian, N. S., McCoy, S. I., Balkus, J. E. & Wasserheit, J. N. (2010). Weighing the gold in the gold standard: Challenges in HIV prevention research. Editorial Review, *AIDS, 24,* 621–635.

Painter, T. M. (2001). Voluntary counseling and testing for couples: A high-leverage intervention for HIV/AIDS prevention in sub-Saharan Africa. *Social Science & Medicine, 53,* 1397–1411.

Park, A. (2014). The end of AIDS, *Time,* December 1–8, 44–52.

Parker, R. (1996). Empowerment, community mobilization, and social change in the face of HIV/AIDS. *AIDS, 10* (Suppl. 3), S27–S31.

———. (2002). The global HIV/AIDS pandemic, structural inequalities, and the politics of international health. *American Journal of Public Health, 92,* 343–346.

———. (2011). Grassroots activism, civil society mobilization, and the politics of the global HIV/AIDS epidemic. *Brown Journal of World Affairs, 17,* 21–27.

Parkhurst, J. O. (2005). The response to HIV/AIDS and the construction of national legitimacy: Lessons from Uganda. *Development and Change, 36,* 571–590.

———. (2008). 'What worked?': The evidence challenges in determining the causes of HIV prevalence decline. *AIDS Education & Prevention, 20,* 275–283.

———. (2012). HIV prevention, structural change and social values: The need for an explicit normative approach. *Journal of the International AIDS Society, 15* (Suppl. 1), 17367.

Patton, C. (2002), *Globalizing AIDS.* Minneapolis and London: University of Minnesota Press.

Paiva, V. (2003). Without magical solutions: HIV and AIDS prevention as a process of psychosocial emancipation. *Divulgação em Saúde Para Debate, 27,* 58–69.

Persson, A. (2010). Reflections on the Swiss Consensus Statement in the context of qualitative interviews with heterosexuals living with HIV. *AIDS Care, 22,* 1487–1492.

Persson, A., Brown, G., McDonald, A. & Korner, H. (2014). Transmission and prevention of HIV among heterosexual populations in Australia. *AIDS Education & Prevention, 26,* 245–255.

Pickles, M., Boily, M-C., Vickerman, P., Lowndes, C. M., Moses, S., Blanchard, J. F. ... Alary, M. (2013). Assessment of the population-level effectiveness of the Avahan HIV-prevention programme in South India: a preplanned, causal-pathway-based modelling analysis. *The Lancet Global Health, 1,* e289–e299.

Piot, P., Quinn, T. C. & Taleman, H. (1984). Acquired immunodeficiency syndrome in a heterosexual population in Zaire. *The Lancet, 2,* 65–69.

Polk, B. F. (1985). Female-to-male transmission of AIDS (letter). *Journal of the American Medical Association, 254,* 3177–3178.

Potterat, J. J., Phillips, L. & Muth, J. B. (1987). Lying to military physicians about risk factors for HIV infections (letter). *Journal of the American Medical Association, 257,* 1727.

Potts, M., Halperin, D. T., Kirby, D., Swidler, A., Marseille, E., Klausner, J. D. ... Walsh, J. (2008). Reassessing HIV prevention. *Science*, *320*, 749–750.

Prestage, G., Brown, G., Down, I., Jin, F. & Hurley, M. (2013). 'It's hard to know what is a risky or not a risky decision': Gay men's beliefs about risk during sex. *AIDS and Behavior*, *17*, 1352–1361.

Putnam, R. (2000). *Bowling Alone: The Collapse and Revival of American Community*. New York: Simon and Schuster.

Race, K. (2012). Framing responsibility: HIV, biomedical research and the performativity of the law. *Journal of Bioethical Inquiry*, *9*, 327–338.

———. (2014a). The difference practice makes: Evidence, articulation and affect in HIV Prevention. *AIDS Education & Prevention*, *26*, 256–266.

———. (2014b). Speculative pragmatism and intimate arrangements: Online hook up devices in gay life. *Culture, Health & Sexuality*, *17*, 496–511.

———. (2015). Party 'n' Play: Online hook-up devices and the emergence of PNP practices among gay men. *Sexualities*, *18*, 253–275.

———. (2016). Reluctant objects: Sexual pleasure as a problem of HIV biomedical prevention. *GLQ: A Journal of Lesbian and Gay Studies*, *22*, 1–31.

Reproductive Health Matters Editorial (2000). Efficacy of voluntary counseling and testing for HIV in reducing risk, *Reproductive Health Matters*, *18*, 176–177.

Reynolds, R. (2007). *What Happened to Gay Life?* Sydney: UNSW Press.

Rijsdijk, L. E., Lie, R., Bos, A. E. R., Leerlooijer, J. N. & Kok, G. (2013). Sexual and reproductive health and rights: Implications for comprehensive sex education among young people in Uganda. *Sex Education*, *13*, 409–422.

Rodger, A., Bruun, T., Cambiano, V., Vernazza, P., Estrada, P., Van Lunzen, J. ... Lundgren, J. for the PARTNER Study Group (2014). HIV transmission risk through condomless sex if HIV +ve partner on suppressive ART: PARTNER study. Paper presented at the 21st Conference on Retroviruses and Opportunistic Infections, Boston.

Rodrigues-Garcia, R., Wilson, D. & York, N. (Eds.) (2013). Effects of investing in communities on HIV/AIDS outcomes. *AIDS Care*, 25 (Suppl. 1).

Rosengarten, M. (2009). *HIV Interventions: Biomedicine and the Traffic between Information and Flesh*. Seattle: University of Washington Press.

Rosengarten, M., Race, K. & Kippax, S. (2000). *'Touch Wood, Everything will be OK': Gay Men's Understandings of Clinical Markers in Sexual Practice*. Sydney: National Centre in HIV Social Research, University of New South Wales.

Rowe, M. & Dowsett, G. (2008). Sex, love, friendship, belonging and place. *Culture, Health & Sexuality*, *10*, 329–344.

Ruxrungtham, K., Brown, T. & Phanuphak, P. (2004). HIV/AIDS in Asia. *The Lancet*, *364*, 69–82.

Saxton, P., Dickson, N., McAllister, S., Sharples, K. & Hughes, A. (2011). Increase in HIV diagnoses among men who have sex with men in New Zealand from a stable low period. *Sexual Health*, *8*, 311–318.

Schein, E. H. (1958). The Chinese indoctrination program for prisoners of war: A study of attempted 'brainwashing'. In *Readings in Social Psychology* (3rd Edition), edited by E. E. Maccoby, T. M. Newcombe & E. L. Hartley, 311–334. London: Methuen & Co.

Schwartländer, B., Stover, J., Hallett, T., Atun, R., Avila, C., Gouws, E. ... on behalf of the UNAIDS Investment Framework Study Group (2011). Towards an improved investment approach for an effective response to HIV/AIDS. *The Lancet*, *377*, 2031–2041.

Seckinelgin, H. (2008). *International Politics of HIV/AIDS: Local Diseases – Local Pain*. London & New York: Routledge.

Seeley, J. (2015). *HIV and East Africa: Thirty Years in the Shadow of an Epidemic*. London: Routledge.

Seeley, J., Watts, C., Kippax, S., Russell, S., Heise, L. & Whiteside, A. (2012). Addressing the structural drivers of HIV: A luxury or necessity for programmes. *Journal of the International AIDS Society, 15* (Suppl. 1), 17397.

Segal, H. A., (1954). Initial psychiatric findings of recently repatriated prisoners of war. *American Journal of Psychiatry, 111*, 358–363.

Sen, A. (1993). Capability and well-being. In *The Quality of Life*, edited by M. Nussbaum & A. Sen, 30–53. New York: Oxford Clarendon Press.

———. (2005). Human rights and capabilities. *Journal of Human Development, 6*, 151–166.

Shallice, T. (1972). The Ulster depth interrogation techniques and their relation to sensory deprivation research, *Cognition, 1*, 385–405.

Sherr, L., Lopman, B., Kakowa, M., Dube, S., Chawira, G., Nyamukapa, C., Oberzaucher, N., Cremin, I. & Gregson, S. (2007). Voluntary counselling and testing: Uptake, impact on sexual behaviour, and HIV incidence in a rural Zimbabwean cohort. *AIDS, 21*, 851–860.

Shisana, O., Rehle, T, Simbayi, L. C., Zuma, K., Jooste, S., Zungu, N., Labadarios, D., Onoya, D. … Wabiri, N. (2014). *South African National HIV Prevalence, Incidence and Behaviour Survey, 2012*. Cape Town: HSRC Press.

Singh, S., Darroch, J. E. & Bankole, A. (2004). A, B and C in Uganda: The Roles of Abstinence, Monogamy and Condom Use in HIV Decline. *Reproductive Health Matters, 12*, 129–135.

Simms, B. (2013). World Bank: Harnessing civil society expertise in undertaking and disseminating research findings. *AIDS Care*, 25 (Suppl. 1), S1–S3.

Slutkin, G., Okware, S., Naamara, W., Sutherland, D., Flanagan, D., Carael, M., Blas, E., Delay, P. & Tarantola, D. (2006). How Uganda reversed its HIV epidemic. *AIDS and Behavior, 10*, 351–361.

Smart, B. (2003). *Economy, Culture and Society*. Buckingham: Open University Press.

Smith, D. J. (2014). *AIDS Doesn't Show its Face: Inequality, Morality and Social Change in Nigeria*. Chicago: University of Chicago Press.

Smith, G. (2005). *Bugger Me! The Civilizing of a Perversion*. (Unpublished PhD thesis). University of New South Wales, Sydney, Australia.

Somaini, B. (2012). The early response to AIDS in Switzerland: A personal view. *Journal of Public Health Policy, 33*, 301–308.

Somaini, B. & Grob, P. (2012). How and why AIDS changed drug policy in Switzerland. *Journal of Public Health Policy, 33*, 317–324.

Sommer, M. & Parker, R. (Eds.) (2013). *Structural Approaches in Public Health*. London: Routledge.

South African National AIDS Council (2012). *Global AIDS Response Progress Report 2012*. National Department of Health and the Research, Monitoring and Evaluation Technical Task Team of the South African National AIDS Council.

Stephenson, N. & Kippax, S. (1999). Minding the gap: Subjectivity and sexuality research, in W. Maiers, B. Bayer, B. Duarte Esgalhado, R. Jorna & E. Schraube (Eds.), *Challenges to Theoretical Psychology*, 383–400. Ontario: Captus Press Inc.

Stephenson, N. & Kippax, S. (2006). Transfiguring relations: Theorising political change in the everyday. *Theory & Psychology, 16*, 391–415.

Stillwaggon, E. (2009). Complexity, cofactors and the failure of AIDS policy in Africa. *Journal of the International AIDS Society, 12*, 1–9.

Stoneburner, R. L., Low-Beer, D., Tembo, G. S., Mertens, G. E. & Asiimwe-Okiror, G. (1996). Human immunodeficiency virus infection dynamics in East Africa deduced from surveillance. *American Journal of Epidemiology, 12*, 435–449.

Stoneburner, R. & Low-Beer, D. (2004). Population-level HIV declines and behavioural risk avoidance in Uganda. *Science, 304*, 714–718.

Sturke, R., Harmston, C., Simonds, R. J. Mofenson, L. M., Siberry, G. K., Watts, D. H., McIntyre, J., Anand, N., Guay, L., Castor, D., Brouwers, P. & Nagel, J. D. (2014). A multi-disciplinary approach to implementation science: The NIH-PEPFAR PMTCT Implementation Science Alliance. *Journal of Acquired Immune Deficiency Syndrome, 67* (Suppl. 2), S163–S167.

Suarez, T. & Miller, J. (2001). Negotiating risks in context: a perspective on unprotected anal intercourse and barebacking among men who have sex with men: Where do we go from here? *Archives of Sexual Behavior, 30*, 287–300.

Sullivan, P. S., Hamouda, O., Delpech, V., Geduld, J. E., Prejean, J., Semaile, C. ... Annecy MSM Epidemiology Study Group. (2009). Reemergence of the HIV epidemic among men who have sex with men in North America, Western Europe, and Australia, 1996–2005. *Annals of Epidemiology, 19*, 423–431.

Sullivan, P. S., Jones, J. S. & Baral, S. D. (2014). The global north: HIV epidemiology in high-income countries. *Current Opinion in HIV and AIDS, 9*, 199–205.

Swidler, A. (2009). Responding to AIDS in Sub-Saharan Africa: Culture, institutions and health. In *Successful Stories: How Institutions and Culture Affect Health*, edited by P. Hall & M. Lamont, 128–150. Cambridge: Cambridge University Press.

Tanser, F., Barnighausen, T., Graspa, E., Zaidi, J. & Newell, M.-L. (2013). High coverage of ART associated with decline in risk of HIV acquisition in rural KwaZulu-Natal, South Africa. *Science, 339*, 966–971.

Tarrow, S. (1996). *Power in Movement.* Cambridge: Cambridge University Press.

The Voluntary HIV-1 Counseling and Efficacy Study group (2000). Efficacy of voluntary HIV-1 counseling and testing in individuals and couples in Kenya, Tanzania, and Trinidad: A randomized control trial, *The Lancet, 356*, 103–112.

Thomas-Slayter, B. P. & Fisher, W. F. (2011). Social capital and AIDS-resilient communities: Strengthening the AIDS response. *Global Public Health, 6* (Suppl. 3), S323–S343.

Thigpen, M. C., Kebaabetswe, P. M., Paxton, L. A. (2012). Antiretroviral pre-exposure prophylaxis for heterosexual transmission in Botswana. *New England Journal of Medicine, 367*, 423–434.

Thornton, R. J. (2008). *Unimagined Community: Sex, Networks, and AIDS in Uganda and South Africa.* Berkeley and Los Angeles: University of California Press.

Triechler, P. (1987). AIDS, homophobia, and biomedical discourse: An epidemic of signification. *Cultural Studies, 1*, 263–305.

Turan, J., Bukusi, E., Onono, M., Holzemer, W., Miller, S. & Cohen, C. (2011). HIV/AIDS Stigma and Refusal of HIV Testing Among Pregnant Women in Rural Kenya: Results from the MAMAS Study. *AIDS and Behavior, 15*, 1111–1120.

Uganda AIDS Commission (2010). *UNGASS Country Progress Response Progress Uganda, March, 2010.* Kampala: Uganda AIDS Commission.

———. (2011). *National Priority Action Plan 2011/2012–2012/2013. March, 2011.* Kampala: Uganda AIDS Commission.

———. (2012). *Global AIDS Response Progress Report: Uganda Jan., 2010–Dec., 2012.* Kampala: Uganda AIDS Commission.

———. (2014). *2013 Uganda HIV and AIDS Country Progress Report.* Kampala: Uganda AIDS Commission.

Uganda Bureau of Statistics (UBOS) & ORC Macro (2001). *Uganda Demographic and Health Survey 2000–2001*. Calverton, MD: UBOS and ORC Macro.

Uganda Bureau of Statistics (UBOS) & Macro International Inc. (2007). *Uganda Demographic and Health Survey 2006*. Calverton, MD: UBOS and Macro International Inc.

Uganda Bureau of Statistics (UBOS) & ICF International Inc. (2012). *Uganda Demographic and Health Survey 2011*. Kampala and Calverton, MD: UBOS and ICF International Inc.

UNAIDS (1999). *Best Practice Collection: Trends in HIV Incidence and Prevalence: Natural Course of the Epidemic or Results of Behavioural Change?* Geneva: UNAIDS.

———. (2000). *Report on the Global HIV/AIDS Epidemic*. Geneva: UNAIDS.

———. (2005). *Intensifying HIV Prevention: A UNAIDS Policy Position Paper*. Geneva: UNAIDS.

———. (2006). *Report on the Global AIDS Epidemic*. Geneva: UNAIDS.

———. (2011). *UNAIDS Terminology Guidelines*. Geneva: UNAIDS. Retrieved from http://www.unaids.org/sites/default/files/media_asset/JC2118_terminology-guidelines_en_0.pdf

———. (2012a). *2012 Progress Reports Submitted by Countries*. Retrieved from http://www.unaids.org/en/dataanalysis/knowyourresponse/countryprogressreports/2012countries/#S

———. (2012b). *Together We Will End AIDS*. Geneva: UNAIDS. Retrieved from http://www.unaids.org/en/resources/campaigns/togetherwewillendaids/unaidsreport/

———. (2012c). *UNAIDS Report on the Global AIDS Epidemic 2012*. Geneva: UNAIDS.

———. (2014a). *Fact Sheet 2014*. Geneva: UNAIDS.

———. (2014b). *2014 Progress Reports Submitted by Countries*. Retrieved from http://www.unaids.org/en/dataanalysis/knowyourresponse/countryprogressreports/2014countries

———. (2014c). *Know Your Epidemic*. Retrieved June 3, 2014, from http://www.unaids.org/en/dataanalysis/knowyourepidemic/

Valdiserri, R. (2013). Preventing HIV/AIDS in the United States, 1981–2009: History in the making. In *The New Public Health and STD/HIV Prevention: Personal, Public and Health System Approaches*, edited by S. O. Aral, K. A. Fenton & J. A. Lipshutz, 309–338. New York: Springer.

Van Damme, L., Corneli, A., Ahmed, K., Agot, K., Lombaard, J. & Kapiga, S. for the FEMPrEP Study Group (2012). Preexposure prophylaxis for HIV infection among African women. *The New England Journal of Medicine, 367*, 411–422.

Van De Perre, P., Jacobs, D. & Sprecher-Goldberger, S. (1987). The latex condom: An efficient barrier against sexual transmission of AIDS-related viruses. *AIDS, 1*, 49–57.

Van der Straten, A., Van Damme, L., Haberer, J. E. & Bangsberg, D. R. (2012). Unravelling the divergent results of pre-exposure prophylaxis trials for HIV prevention. *AIDS, 26*, F13–F19.

Van de Ven, P., Kippax, S., Knox, S., Prestage, G. & Crawford, J. (1999). HIV treatments optimism and sexual behaviour among gay men in Sydney and Melbourne. *AIDS, 13*, 2289–2294.

Van de Ven, P., Prestage, G., Crawford, J., Grulich, A. & Kippax, S. (2000). Sexual risk behaviour increases and is associated with HIV optimism among HIV-negative and HIV-positive gay men in Sydney over the 4 year period to February. *AIDS, 14*, 2951–2953.

Van de Ven, P., Rawstorne, P., Nakamura, T., Crawford, J. & Kippax, S. (2002). HIV treatments optimism is associated with unprotected anal intercourse with regular and with casual partners among Australian gay and homosexually active men. *International Journal of STD & AIDS, 13*, 181–183.

Van de Ven, P., Rawstorne, P., Treloar C. & Richters, J. (Eds.) (2003). *HIV/AIDS, Hepatitis C and Related Diseases in Australia: Annual Report of Behaviour.* Sydney: National Centre in HIV Social Research, UNSW.

Van de Ven, P., Murphy, D., Hull, P., Prestage, G., Batrouney, C. & Kippax, S. (2004). Risk management and harm reduction among gay men in Sydney. *Critical Public Health, 14*, 361–376.

Van de Ven, P., Mao, L., Fogarty, A., Rawstorne, P., Crawford, J., Prestage, G. ... Kippax, S. (2005). Undetectable viral load is associated with sexual risk taking in HIV serodiscordant gay couples in Sydney. *AIDS, 19*, 179–184.

Van Griensven, F., de Lind van Wijngaarden, J. W., Baral, S. & Grulich, A. (2009). The global epidemic of HIV infection among men who have sex with men. *Current Opinion in HIV and AIDS, 4*, 300–307.

Van Sighem, A., Vidondo, B., Glass, T. R., Bucher, H. C., Vernazza, P., Gebhardt, M. ... Low, N. & the Swiss Cohort Study (2012). Resurgence of HIV infection among men who have sex with men in Switzerland: Mathematical modeling study. *PLOS, One 7*, e44819.

Vermund, S. H., Tique, J. A., Cassell, H. M., Pask, M. E., Ciampa, P. J. & Audet, C. M. (2013). Translation of biomedical prevention strategies for HIV: Prospects and pitfalls. *Journal of Acquired Immune Deficiency Syndrome, 63* (Suppl.1), S12–S25.

Vernazza, P., Hirschel, B. & Bernasconi, E. (2008). Les personnes seropositives suivant un TAR efficace ne transmettant pas le VIH pat voie sexuelle. *Bulletin de Medicins Suisses, 89*, 5.

Vico, G. (2002). *The First New Science* (L. Pompa, trans.). Cambridge: Cambridge University Press. (Original work published 1725).

Vincent, R. & Miskelly, C. (2010). Measuring social and structural change for HIV prevention. Paper presented at the Think Tank on Evaluation of HIV Prevention, Wilson Park, Sussex, UK.

Waldby, C. (1996). *AIDS and the Body Politic: Biomedicine and Sexual Difference.* London: Routledge.

Waldby, C., Kippax, S. & Crawford, J. (1993). Cordon Sanitaire: 'clean' and 'unclean' women in the AIDS discourse of young men. In *AIDS: Facing the Second Decade*, edited by P. Aggleton, P. Davies & G. Hart, 29–39. London: Falmer Press.

Waldby, C., Kippax, S. & Crawford, J. (1995). Epidemiological knowledge and discriminatory practice: AIDS and the social relations of biomedicine. *Australian and New Zealand Journal of Sociology, 31*, 1–14.

Ward, J., Costello-Czok, M., Willis, J., Saunders, M. & Shannon, C. (2014). So far, so good: Maintenance of prevention is required to stem HIV incidence in Aboriginal and Torres Strait Islanders in Australia. *AIDS Education & Prevention, 26*, 267–279.

Weeks, J. (1998). The Sexual Citizen. *Theory, Culture & Society, 15*, 35–52.

Wellings, K., Collumbien, M., Slaymaker, E., Singh, S., Hodges, Z., Patel, D. & Bajos, N. (2006). Sexual behaviour in context: A global perspective. *The Lancet, 368*, 1706–1728.

Weinhardt, L. S., Carey, M. P., Johnson, B. T. & Bickham, N. L. (1999). Effects of HIV counseling and testing on sexual risk behavior: A meta-analytic review of published research, 1985–1997. *American Journal of Public Health, 89*, 1397–1405.

Westercamp, N., Agot, K., Jaoko, W. & Bailey, R. (2014). Risk compensation following male circumcision: Results from a two-year prospective cohort study of recently circumcised and uncircumcised men in Nyanza Province, Kenya. *AIDS and Behavior, 18*, 1764–1775.

Whiteside, A. & Strauss, M. (2014). The end of AIDS: Possibility or pipe dream? A tale of transitions. *African Journal of AIDS Research, 13*, 101–108.

WHO (2012). *Global Monitoring Framework and Strategy for the Global Plan Towards the Elimination of New HIV Infections Among Children by 2015 and Keeping Their Mothers Alive.* Geneva: WHO.

————. (2013a). *Global Update on HIV Treatment 2013: Results, Impact and Opportunities, WHO Report in Partnership with UNICEF and UNAIDS, June 2013.* Geneva: WHO.

————. (2013b). *Consolidated Guidelines on the Use of Antiretroviral Drugs for Treating and Preventing HIV Infection: Recommendations for a Public Health Approach, June 2013.* Geneva: WHO.

————. (2014). *HIV/AIDS, Mother to Child Transmission.* Retrieved from http://www.who.int/hiv/topics/mtct/en/

Williams, G. H. (2003). The determinants of health: Structure, context and agency. *Sociology of Health & Illness, 25*, 131–154.

Wilson, D. & Halperin, D. T. (2008). 'Know your epidemic, know your response': A useful approach, if we get it right. *The Lancet, 372*, 423–426.

Wilson, D. P. (2012). HIV treatment as prevention: Natural experiments highlight limits of antiretroviral treatment as HIV prevention. *PLoS Medicine, 9*, e1001231.

Wilson, D. P., Law, M., Grulich, A., Cooper, D. & Kaldor, J. (2008). Relation between HIV viral load and infectiousness: A model-based analysis. *The Lancet, 372*, 314–320.

Wilson, D. P., Jin, F., Jansson, J., Zablotska, I. & Grulich, A. (2010). Infectiousness of HIV-infected men who have sex with men in the era of highly active antiretroviral therapy. *AIDS, 24*, 2420–2421.

Wit, J. de, Mao, L., Holt, M. & Treloar, C. (2013). *HIV/AIDS, Hepatitis and Sexually Transmissible Infections in Australia: Annual Report of Trends in Behaviour 2013* (Monograph 6/2013). Sydney: Centre for Social Research in Health, University of New South Wales.

Wit, J. de, Mao, L., Adam, P. & Treloar, C. (Eds.) (2014). *HIV/AIDS, Hepatitis and Sexually Transmissible Infections in Australia: Annual Report of Trends in Behaviour 2014* (Monograph). Sydney: Centre for Social Research in Health, University of New South Wales.

Woolcock, M. (2001). The place of social capital in understanding social and economic outcomes. *Canadian Journal of Policy Research, 2*, 66–88.

Zablotska, I., Crawford, J., Imrie, J., Prestage, G., Jin, F., Grulich, A. & Kippax, S. (2009). Increases in unprotected anal intercourse with sero-discordant casual partners among HIV-negative gay men in Sydney. *AIDS and Behavior, 13*, 638–644.

Zablotska, I., Prestage, G., Middleton, M., Wilson, D. & Grulich A. (2010). Contemporary HIV diagnoses trends in Australia can be predicted by trends in unprotected anal intercourse among gay men. *AIDS, 24*, 1955–1958.

Zwi, A. & Cabral, A. J. R. (1991). Identifying 'high risk situations' for preventing AIDS. *British Medical Journal, 303*, 1527–1529.

INDEX

www.ingramcontent.com/pod-product-compliance
Lightning Source LLC
Chambersburg PA
CBHW020000290326
41935CB00007B/247